Multiple Sclerosis: Psychosocial and Vocational Interventions

Multiple Sclerosis: Psychosocial and Vocational Interventions

Robert T. Fraser, Ph.D., C.R.C.

David C. Clemmons, Ph.D., C.R.C.

Francie Bennett, M.S.W.

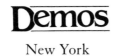

New York

Library of Congress Cataloging-in-Publication Data

Made in the United States of America

Supported by Grant #315-96 of the Education and Training Foundation, Paralyzed Veterans of America and limited partial support of the University of Washington Multiple Sclerosis Rehabilitation Research and Training Center (NIDRR grant #H133B9800017) and Department of Neurology.

This book is dedicated to the thousands of individuals with MS who struggle daily for vocational and independent living, self-sufficiency, and the rehabilitation counseling/allied health personnel who assist them in this challenge.

Contents

Appendix A
US Department of Labor Statement of

Appendix B

Appendix C

Appendix D
National Multiple Sclerosis Society

Appendix E

Preface

This book is an outgrowth of vocational rehabilitation counselor training conducted by the authors in the states of
Washington, Alaska, Montana, Idaho, and Oregon. Feedback from
the counselor attendees helped to refine the book. It will be helpful to
vocational rehabilitation counselors and to all members of the health
care team concerned about the psychosocial status of their clients with
multiple sclerosis.

The first section is a broad-based medical overview of the course
of the MS disease process, its diagnosis and symptomatology, medical
treatments, and rehabilitation. This is followed by a discussion of
neuropsychological concerns, including concepts of importance in
vocational rehabilitation and the specific cognitive and related impairments that are characteristic of MS and that cause vocational difficulties. Subsequent sections are a review of vocational rehabilitation
interventions that focus on assessment and rehabilitation planning, and
by a review of psychosocial issues and interventions that deals with a
wide range of issues that affect the family and community.

The book is designed to be used as a basic training text for an
individual counselor or health professional seeking to learn more
about MS vocational rehabilitation or psychosocial adjustment and
neuropsychology. It can also be used as the core material for training

groups. Case studies are included as small group discussion training tools.

Robert T. Fraser, Ph.D.
David C. Clemmons, Ph.D.
Francie Bennett, M.S.W.

Acknowledgments

Our deep appreciation is extended to the Education and Training Foundation of the Paralyzed Veterans of America (Grant #315-96) for the support of this book's development, its accompanying videos, and the expenses incurred in the training of approximately 250 state agency vocational rehabilitation counselors across five states. Ms. Patricia Armstrong of the Foundation, our liaison, was particularly supportive and patient in our completion of this project. The first two authors are currently involved in vocational rehabilitation research activity through the University of Washington MS Rehabilitation Research and Training Center grant as supported by the National Institute of Disability and Rehabilitation Research (NIDRR). Appreciation is extended to NIDRR and Dr. George Kraft, Director of the Center, for this opportunity and partial support of the book's completion. Our special thanks to Ms. Kai Martin for her preparation of this manuscript—couldn't have done it without you Kai.

About the Authors

Robert T. Fraser, Ph.D., C.R.C. served as the principle director for this project of which this book is a byproduct. He is a licensed rehabilitation psychologist counselor, a certified vocational rehabilitation counselor, and a professor within the University of Washington Departments of Neurology, joint with Neurological Surgery and Rehabilitation Medicine. He has directed the University of Washington's Project With Industry since 1979 and received a number of grant awards from the Rehabilitation Services Administration, the National Institute of Disability and Rehabilitation Research, the National Institutes of Health, the Epilepsy Foundation of America, and other sources. He has been author or co-author of more than 80 publications and co-edited two new books: *Traumatic Brain Injury Rehabilitation: Practical Vocational, Neuropsychological, and Psychotherapy Interventions* with Dr. Clemmons and *Comprehensive Care for People with Epilepsy*. Dr. Fraser is a past president of Division 22, Rehabilitation Psychology of the American Psychological Association and served on the Board and Professional Advisory Boards of the Epilepsy Foundation of America.

David C. Clemmons, Ph.D., C.R.C. is a research scientist within the Department of Neurology and Director of Vocational Services for the Epilepsy Center. He is a licensed rehabilitation psychologist, a certified vocational rehabilitation counselor, and an investigator or co-investigator on seven federal grants within the last 12 years. Dr. Clemmons has been the coordinating representative for the Project With Industry to the King County Multiple Sclerosis Association. Dr. Clemmons, in addition to the MS vocational rehabilitation training grant, has led up to three-day training programs in traumatic brain injury and epilepsy rehabilitation by himself and with Dr. Fraser at numerous sites around the country (e.g., The Rehabilitation Institute of Chicago, the Minot State University in North Dakota, the Ontario Brain Injury Association, the States of Montana and Idaho Divisions of Vocational Rehabilitation, etc.). In addition to co-editorship work with Dr. Fraser, he has been lead director of a traumatic brain injury rehabilitation video series with a counseling or psychotherapy emphasis currently distributed by CRC Press.

Francie Bennett, MSW is a Washington state Licensed Independent Social Worker. She received her Masters from the University of Washington, School of Social Work and is an affiliate faculty of that school. Bennett is a psychotherapist, trainer and consultant in the Seattle, Washington area. In addition to providing trainings in five states on this book's topic, she has also served as an Executive Director of a non-profit services agency and as a social worker within the MS community. She has provided counseling and assessments, as an independent contractor, to Washington state vocational rehabilitation participants. Bennett enjoys working with a broad range of people and issues within her private practice.

For purposes of training requests, groups seeking a comprehensive training package as presented by the authors in the book can contact Drs. Fraser or Clemmons at the University of Washington Department of Neurology-Epilepsy Center, Harborview Medical Center, Box 359744, Seattle, Washington 98104, (206) 341-4545, fax (206) 731-6088, email rfraser@u.washington.edu or clemmons@u.washington.edu. If training is desired solely in relation to psychosocial assessments, counseling, and/or case management, Ms. Bennett can be contacted directly at (206) 440-9706, email fkbennett2000@yahoo.com. If training is sought specific to vocational rehabilitation or neuropsychology areas, again contact can be made with Drs. Fraser or Clemmons as above. All book profits will be used by the authors to support further training efforts.

Multiple Sclerosis: Psychosocial and Vocational Interventions

Multiple Sclerosis— A Medical Overview

David C. Clemmons, Ph.D., C.R.C.

Multiple sclerosis (MS) is one of a number of central nervous system (CNS) conditions termed demyelinating diseases. Myelin is a fatty substance that is produced by special Schwann cells within the CNS and coats CNS neurons. Myelin serves both to protect the nerve cells and to promote the efficient transmission of electrical impulses along the axons of nerve cells. Many congenital disorders such as phenylketonuria and Tay-Sachs syndrome affect the development of myelin sheathing early in life. Other factors, such as decreased blood flow and the presence of toxins, may also degrade myelin, either temporarily or permanently. When myelin loss is extensive and permanent, a degeneration of the neurons themselves may occur, which can be permanent. Because the CNS damage in demyelinating diseases occurs primarily in the so-called *white matter*, the connecting cells beneath the cerebral cortex, some of these conditions are also grouped as *subcortical dementias*.

Multiple sclerosis is the most common of the demyelinating diseases. It is a CNS disorder of slow and often uneven progression. It is characterized by multiple demyelinated (sclerotic) regions that may occur either in the brain itself, in the brain stem, or in the spinal cord. Symptoms of MS may vary greatly from individual to individual, and the condition is often characterized by periodic remissions and exacerbations, sometimes separated by many months or even years.

1

The prevalence of MS is strongly associated with geographic location. It may be as high as 1:2,000 in the northern latitudes, decreasing to 1:10,000 in the tropics. It appears to be a condition that primarily affects those of northern European ancestry, although exclusion from this group does not confer immunity. There is some increased incidence within families, suggesting a possible genetic factor to the condition, and females are more frequently affected than are males, possibly by a factor of two. Multiple sclerosis is diagnosed most frequently between the ages of 20 and 45, although people of any age may be vulnerable. Except in relatively rare cases, life span is not greatly affected (Poser et al., 1984).

Research on MS has not identified a specific cause for the condition, and effective cures have not been developed. Once diagnosed, MS is considered a chronic condition. Much evidence suggests an etiology characterized by immune system dysfunction, possibly triggered by a viral agent, in a genetically predisposed population.

Disease Course

The course of MS generally falls into one of three groups: a relapsing-remitting, a primary progressive, or a secondary progressive pattern. There presently exists considerable speculation as to whether this typology adequately describes MS and whether the proposed subtypes are not in actuality superficial manifestations of a similar disease process. This is an area of continuing research and speculation. In each of these categories, the condition exists chronically, often for decades. Figure I-1 shows the disease pattern of the various MS subtypes.

Relapsing-Remitting Multiple Sclerosis

Relapsing-remitting MS is characterized by acute symptoms, or exacerbations, followed by periods of full or partial recovery or remissions. The period between exacerbations is free from obvious progression of the disease, although some sources suggest that the condition continues to progress on a subclinical level, a situation in which the patient continues to lose residual capacity due to formation of MS lesions without

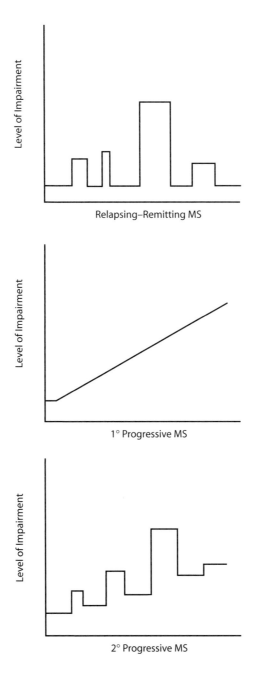

FIGURE I-1 Various Multiple Sclerosis subtypes.

suffering immediate loss of function. The time between remissions and exacerbations may be considerable, in some cases measured by years. Ultimate vocational function is likely to depend on how fully an individual recovers from exacerbations over time. Some individuals lose little or no functioning over time, with apparently full recovery during remission, whereas others may experience a steady decline in function. The severity of one's MS can be rated on the Expanded Disability Status Scale (Kurtzke, 1983) by the physician or self-rated by the patient.

Primary Progressive Multiple Sclerosis

Primary progressive MS involves a steady progression of the disease process from diagnosis or onset. While there may appear to be some slowing of the progression or minor recovery from symptoms, clear periods of remission do not exist. Primary progressive MS is relatively rare compared with the two other main subtypes, although it is likely to be better represented in special populations, such as referrals to vocational rehabilitation clinics. Loss of functional capacity over time generally is substantial.

Secondary Progressive Multiple Sclerosis

Secondary progressive MS is a subtype that initially presents with a relapsing-remitting pattern but secondarily evolves into a primary progressive pattern. As with primary progressive MS, there generally is a steady decline in medical status over time.

Other Multiple Sclerosis Subtypes

Variations exist in the patterns presented above and are sometimes described as separate entities in the literature. Occasional referral is made to *benign MS*, in which the individual experiences no longitudinal loss of function and little disruption of life functioning during exacerbations, which generally are rare. Some sources report remissions that last for as long as 25 years (Berkow, 1982). On the other end of the spectrum is a less common subtype sometimes referred to as malignant MS, in which medical status rapidly declines, with dramatic overall loss of function. This subtype, which could be conceptualized as a rapidly progressing case of primary progressive MS, ordinarily is fatal within a few years of diagnosis.

Diagnosis and Symptomatology

Because MS is a condition of the CNS, MS lesions may disrupt any aspect of CNS functioning. Early onset may be subtle and insidious, with transient symptoms and little in the way of objective clinical findings. Initial MS symptoms frequently involve fatigue, blurry vision, and tingling or weakness in the extremities. Relapses may occur frequently or may be characterized by a gap of months or years, often with complete recovery between relapses during the initial course of the condition. Differential diagnosis involves the elimination of disease entities with similar initial characteristics, such as lupus, transverse myelitis, or various infectious diseases. Following an initial period, the course of the disease may be variable, and some patients may experience varying deficits in motor control and sensory integrity, as well as changes in mental and emotional status. Diagnosis of MS is enhanced by appreciation for its polyphasic nature (i.e., acute illness followed by recovery) as opposed to many other confounding neurologic illnesses that are not characterized by a cycle of exacerbation and recovery.

The advent of imaging technology, such as magnetic resonance imaging (MRI) and positron emission tomography (PET) scans, has made definitive diagnosis more readily available and accurate over the past decade. Aside from analysis of CNS fluid following spinal tap, MS diagnosis historically has been largely presumptive. Because the sclerotic lesions that characterize MS may occur throughout the CNS, symptomatology may vary greatly from patient to patient, often causing complex and diverse symptoms. Although symptoms are theoretically dependent on the location and number of CNS lesions, imaging technology has only recently developed the sophistication and sensitivity to begin to explore this relationship empirically. MRI technology also has the advantage of being noninvasive.

Another aid in the diagnosis of MS is the *evoked visual potential* (EVP) procedure. This procedure involves providing photic stimulation to a patient who is being monitored by electroencephalography in such a manner that the speed of the visual signal from the optic nerve to the occipital lobes may be determined. Deviations from the previously determined normal speed of transmission allows the inference of lesions in this pathway. Finally, a lumbar puncture procedure has traditionally been a diagnostic strategy in MS diagnosis. This involves inserting a needle into the spinal column and withdrawing a small amount of cerebral spinal fluid, which is then analyzed for the presence of antibodies suggesting MS. With the increased use of MRI technology, lumbar puncture is frequently not the first choice of diagnostic strategy.

The most common MS symptoms are listed here under the following categories: emotional/psychological, motor, sensory, autonomic, and cognitive. Although these areas are treated as separate entities in this section, expressed symptoms frequently result from overlapping difficulties in a number of these areas.

Emotional and Psychological Symptoms

Emotional and psychological symptomatology in MS may be due to changes directly attributable to the disease process (i.e., the impact of sclerotic lesions on neural networks) or to a patient's reaction to the course of the disease process (i.e., reactive depression, psychosomatic illnesses). Depending on the lesion site and total lesion load, significant disease-related emotional concerns are not uncommon in MS. Emotional lability, with spells of crying or laughter, may occur.

TABLE I-1.   Emotional/Psychological MS Symptoms

- Organic: — Lability
            — Euphoria
- Reactive: — Depression
            — Fear
            — Anxiety

Euphoria, a technical term suggesting an exaggerated feeling of well-being, may be present (see Table I-1). These concerns are treated in more detail in Section IV.

Motor Symptoms

When sclerotic plaques involve neurons associated with motor function, fatigue, muscle weakness, and dyscoordination may occur (see Table I-2). Disturbance of gait is a hallmark concern of motor function in MS, and a combination of muscular weakness and poor coordination may produce a characteristically wide and stumbling gait. Many people with advanced disability need to use a cane, a walkers, or a wheelchairs. Muscular weakness and dyscontrol in the upper extremities are also common and, when combined with tremor and spasticity, make fine motor activity such as handwriting, typing, and similar activities quite difficult. Unfortunately, some of the tremor seen in MS is intention tremor (i.e., a tremor exacerbated by attempting to use the muscle group in question). This is contrasted with static tremor (i.e., a tremor when muscle groups are at rest), which may also be present.

Sensory Symptoms

There are a number of sensory concerns that can be associated with MS (see Table I-3). A common sensory symptom involves changes in vision. Although total blindness is rarely a sequela of MS, a decrease in visual acuity, sometimes to the point where legal blindness is an issue, occurs in a significant minority of patients. Some patients begin

---

TABLE I-2.   Motor (Muscle) MS Symptoms

- Disturbance of gait
- Weakness
- Dyscoordination
- Tremor
- Decreased fine motor control

TABLE I-3.   Sensory MS Symptoms

- Visual anomalies
- Decreased tactile sensation (may be transitory)
- Difficulties with balance/proprioception
- Pain
- Sexual dysfunction in women and men

with a transient and frequently unilateral blindness that resolves over a period of weeks or months. This concern, due to *optic neuritis*, is only one of many possible ocular changes in MS. Partial atrophy of the optic nerve, narrowing of the visual field, double vision, and decreased visual acuity all are possible sequelae of MS.

With respect to tactile sensation, a blunting of sensation and numbness are common, often localized, and possibly transient. Complete loss of tactile sensation is rare, with partial numbness or tingling of affected areas being the rule. Pain, especially in advanced disease, may be a significant component of sensory disruption, as in *Lhermitte's syndrome*, in which the patient experiences a sensation of electrical tingling or frank pain in the arms or back when flexing muscles of the shoulder girdle. Difficulties with balance and proprioception also may occur and may constitute safety issues when walking, using machinery, or working in a potentially dangerous physical environment.

Autonomic Symptoms

As with sensory and motor signs, initial autonomic symptomatology may be subtle and transient and can vary greatly among patients (see Table I-4). Urogenital symptoms may include sexual impotence in

TABLE I-4.   Autonomic MS Symptoms

- Retention of urine
- Bowel and bladder incontinence
- Male impotence

men, difficulty in urination, and partial retention of urine. Bowel and bladder incontinence may exist, especially in advanced cases. Other autonomic symptoms (i.e., changes in heart rate, blood pressure, etc.) are not manifested in MS.

Additional Physical Functional Limitations

Multiple sclerosis presents a number of other medically related concerns that overlap the schema presented above and are often encountered in MS vocational rehabilitation (see Table I-5). These include difficulties with physical fatigue, sensitivity to heat, and difficulties with follow-through and continuity of activity related to the cyclic nature of the disease.

Fatigue

Physical fatigue is a common concern for people with MS and a very common issue with MS vocational rehabilitation clients. Because of the nature of the disease, MS-related fatigue may not be as alleviated by rest or sleep as is the case with the general population. The physical stamina required for a traditional eight-hour shift may be beyond the endurance of many vocational rehabilitation clients with the disability. This is espe-

---

TABLE I-5.   Additional Physical MS Symptoms

Fatigue
- Not always remediated by rest
- Exacerbated by inefficiency due to poor motor control
- Interactions with cognitive status
- Interactions with emotional status

Sensitivity to heat
- Lowers efficiency
- May preclude vocational participation periodically
- Large individual variation
- Use of "low-tech" devices such as cooling jackets

---

cially true if one also considers the physical demands on the client with respect to transportation to work, completion of daily chores, and the increased physical burden that may be imposed by difficulty with ambulation and motor control. A desirable work situation for people with these concerns may be one in which a worker could work in intervals or at will. This ideal situation could involve a schedule incorporating helpful rest periods during a day. It could even allow for work to be done over a 24-hour period, maximizing a client's most productive time. Such an employment situation would almost of necessity be home-based. While many clients with MS accommodate their fatigue concerns, the rehabilitation worker should keep in mind that approximating an ideal work situation by minimizing transportation problems or arranging for work situations that allow for rest or break periods will maximize a client's ability to maintain employment. Some people with MS work best with a shift that utilizes their daily hours of optimal functioning or with a shortened workday (e.g., six hours a day). A job share arrangement could be ideal and may result in optimal schedules.

The rehabilitation professional should be aware that there may be a negative interaction between increased fatigue and emotional and psychological status. It should be noted that the "language of fatigue" can also be used to describe depression. Some individuals who begin the day "tired" or who are constantly tired might be assessed for the effects of depression.

Sensitivity to Heat

As with fatigue, sensitivity to heat can significantly reduce the efficiency of the worker with MS. While many people with CNS disease may demonstrate increased sensitivity to heat, people with MS seem to be particularly vulnerable. Although sensitivity to heat should be explored for all vocational rehabilitation clients, there is considerable variation, with some individuals generally being incapacitated by higher temperatures. Heat sensitivity in MS implies not merely discomfort, but also a reduced efficiency, which may be both mental and physical, in some patients. Of concern is summer weather, particularly heat spells, and work sites with poor circulation and temperature control.

A number of "low-tech" strategies for dealing with heat sensitivity exist, many of which incorporate cooling jackets, vests, or collars that may be filled with cool water. These are readily available commercially. Employer accommodations for heat sensitivity may include supplying air-conditioning to the client's work site, reducing job duties outside a controlled environment, resituating the work site away from windows and other heat sources, and similar strategies. As with concerns about fatigue, a desirable accommodation may also include restructuring the work load from a full- to part-time schedule or to a home-based work site.

Cognitive Symptomatology

Significant cognitive change is thought to occur within a range of 42 percent to 63 percent of the general population of people with MS (Rao, 1995) and may be higher in populations such as those seen in specialty clinics and rehabilitation facilities. People with MS who do demonstrate changes in cognitive status may be vulnerable to difficulties with short-term memory, especially retrieval processes, decreased cognitive efficiency and speed of information processing, and difficulties with higher order functions such as abstraction, problem solving, and decision making. Other cognitive concerns, such as difficulty with attention and concentration, disruption in language usage, and so forth, may also occur. Frank dementia ordinarily is not present except in some late-stage illness. The type and intensity of cognitive change varies greatly depending on the individual.

Cognitive symptoms, when present, are appropriately assessed by neuropsychological testing batteries. The strategy in neuropsychological testing is not to simply establish intellectual functioning (via IQ tests or other unidimensional tests of ability) but rather to review a broad spectrum of cognitive functioning. Table I-6 reviews seven areas important to vocational functioning that are often explored by neuropsychological testing, although many people with MS have a more restricted pattern of impairment, as previously referenced. This subject is treated in greater depth in Section II.

TABLE I-6.   Seven Areas Explored in Neuropsychological Testing for Vocational Rehabilitation Counseling

Sensorimotor Ability:
Do the areas of the brain responsible for controlling the body's muscles function efficiently? Does the brain efficiently process input from the sensory organs?

Attention and Concentration:
The ability to attend to individual stimuli. The ability to focus attention on a stimulus in the presence of distractions or for an extended period of time.

Memory:
Visual-spatial memory, verbal memory, long- and short-term memory, incidental memory vs memory for rehearsed or practiced items.

Language Ability:
The ability to understand language and to use language to express ideas.

Spatial Ability:
Ability to deal with two- and three-dimensional formats, perceive part to whole relationships, perceive field-background relationships.

Cognitive Efficiency:
The ability to efficiently perform simultaneous tasks or tasks in the presence of distractors. The ability to screen out extraneous stimuli.

Executive Function:
Abstraction, problem-solving, self-regulation, initiation.

This outline is intended as a model for describing various cognitive abilities important in the vocational rehabilitation of brain-injured persons. The areas listed above are not necessarily independent entities, and may overlap with one another.

Cyclical Nature of Multiple Sclerosis and Interactions Between Symptoms

The presence of MS symptom exacerbations, especially when frequent, presents an especially difficult problem to vocational rehabilitation efforts. As with other CNS concerns, such as stroke or traumatic brain injury, an individual client's potential may best be described not by his or her highest level of functioning at a given time but by an average level of functioning that takes into account many other considerations, such as the impact of stress, fluctuating disability exacerbations, or problems with gait and mobility on work performance. For clients with a multiplicity of symptoms, as well as with clients who have frequent exacerbations, there is likely to be a synergistic interaction between symptoms that may considerably affect employment issues (see Table I-7). Employer accommodations, as discussed throughout this section, may allow the employee to have greater control of work flow. Home-based employment becomes an increasingly desirable option as diverse symptoms become more pressing.

Medical Treatment and Medication

Medications used to treat MS may be separated into two groups: medications used to alter the course of the disease and medications used to treat symptoms. Until the last decade, symptomatic treatment was the only option available, with a variety of tranquilizers, muscle relaxants, and similar agents being used to deal with muscle cramps, difficulty with bowel and bladder functioning, constipation, and so forth. While symptomatic treatment continues to be appropriate, immunosuppressant and immunomodulatory strategies developed in the last decade attempt to change the course of the condition by inhibiting the process of myelin degeneration. This has frequently involved the use of a class of drugs called *corticosteroids*. Corticosteroids currently approved for use in MS include prednisone, the beta interferons (i.e., Betaseron, Avonex, or Rebif), and glatiramer acetate (Copaxone). In relation to intervention, there are a number of arguments that favor one drug over another (i.e., the frequency of exacerbations, etc.) (Bowen, 1999). Presently there are a number of other drugs currently under development—the good news

TABLE I-7   Cyclic Nature of MS Symptoms

- Makes vocational planning difficult
- May decrease overall efficiency
- Interactions with emotional/psychological status

is that this is an area in which gains are being made, and a number of those with MS would profit from a current medication referral. Many people with MS do not know that new medications are available.

In relation to initiating treatment or treating those with a mild form of MS (at time of presentation), there are competing schools of thought. The National Multiple Sclerosis Society currently endorses the view that all patients be treated with a disease-modifying medication because most patients experience increasing disability over time, apparent physical stability does not connote a lack of progressive CNS lessening (or the lack of cognitive loss), damage that can occur is not later reversible, those in early disease stages respond better, and there are no serious medical side effects. Contrarians would point to the inconvenience, cost, and still potential "uncomfortable" side effects of medications (Bowen, 1999).

Rehabilitation

Kraft (1998) reviews a number of rehabilitation principles to improve the functional prognosis for a person with MS. He is an advocate for medication management of spasticity, which he believes is related to fatigue. He recommends medical management of fatigue (e.g., amantadine) but also body cooling and a mild to moderate aerobic exercise program. He recommends other simple interventions for balance (e.g., a cane) and upper limb ataxic tremor problems (e.g., wrist weights). For difficulties with weakness management, he describes the roles of resistive exercise, orthoses (e.g., ankle bracing), and possible electrical stimulation in the shoe or ankle brace to assist in walking. Kraft endorses mastery of a range of rehabilitation strategies that can be particularly useful when employed during disease exacerbations.

Summary

Medical knowledge and treatment of MS is presently experiencing a period of development. New treatment and diagnostic options will likely replace traditional medical practice. For this reason, specific medications and treatment strategies have not been emphasized in depth in this chapter. Rather, a focus has been on the demography of MS and symptomatology that is likely to present functional limitations in a vocational context. Although a complete cure or complete control of MS symptoms does not appear to be probable in the foreseeable future, partial control of MS symptomatology through medical advances does seem likely. At the same time, advances in technology that impact rehabilitation efforts (e.g., voice-activated computer systems) can be expected to maximize residual abilities for this population.

Multiple sclerosis is described herein as a demyelinating disease of the CNS, most frequently occurring between the ages of 20 and 40, and occurring more frequently in women than in men. Although typically a disease of people with northern European ancestry, people of any racial background may contract MS. Because it is a CNS disease, symptomatology may include disruptions in sensory function, motor function, cognition, and/or emotional status. Common symptomatology includes fatigue, visual problems, and difficulties with gait and fine motor function. In vocational rehabilitation contexts, relatively high levels of cognitive and emotional concerns are frequently observed. Multiple sclerosis frequently is characterized by exacerbation of symptomatology followed by periods of remission that may last months or even years. Most people with MS will experience a normal life span, although increasing levels of symptomatology may cause increasing vocational and independent living impairment.

Although a fluctuating medical condition may make assessment for vocational rehabilitation challenging, an attempt should be made to generate a history of past exacerbations and remissions, as well as the present physical and cognitive difficulties, and to develop a "best guess" for future levels of function. Vocational rehabilitation practitioners, especially those who practice outside larger metropolitan areas, should make an attempt to keep abreast of the rapidly changing medical and technical applications relevant to MS vocational rehabilitation to ensure that clients can maximize their potential performance.

References

Berkow, R., ed. (1984). *The Merck manual of diagnosis and therapy*. Merck Sharp & Dohme Research Laboratories, Rahway, NJ, 1354–1357.

Bowen, J. (1999). Medical management of multiple sclerosis. Paper presented at the 18th University of Washington Review Course in Physical Medicine and Rehabilitation, Seattle, Washington.

Kraft, G.H. (1998). Rehabilitation principles for patients with multiple sclerosis. *J Spinal Cord Med* 21(2):117–120.

Kurtzke, J.F. (1983). Rating neurological impairment in multiple sclerosis: An expanded disability status scale (EDSS). *Neurology* 33:1444-52.

Poser et al. (1984). *Merritt's textbook of neurology*, 7th ed. L.P. Rowland (ed.), Lea & Febiger, Philadelphia, 593–615.

Rao, S.M. (1995). Neuropsychology of multiple sclerosis. *Curr Opin Neurol* 8(3):216–20.

Neuropsychological Concerns

David C. Clemmons, Ph.D., C.R.C.

Because multiple sclerosis (MS) is a disease of the central nervous system (CNS), some disruption of cognitive abilities is frequently an important symptom to consider in vocational planning. The incidence and severity of cognitive disruption in MS has historically been underestimated or basically denied. In the past decade, a vast body of growing evidence has implicated significant cognitive dysfunction as an important consideration in providing services to people with MS (Brassington and Marsh, 1998; Grafman et al., 1991; Rao et al., 1991; Arvett et al., 1997). Although many people with MS experience only very mild problems or no difficulties with cognition, there is good reason to believe that the incidence of cognitive difficulties or established brain impairment approximates 45 percent to 65 percent in the general population of people with MS (Rao, 1995). This incidence may be higher in specialized situations, such as medical specialty clinics and vocational rehabilitation programs. It is important to avoid the mistake of assuming that a diagnosis of MS automatically implies significant difficulties in cognitive ability. It is equally important, however, to provide sufficient screening and evaluation to ensure that cognitive difficulties are not overlooked in the development of a rehabilitation plan.

One might expect that a client who has significant cognitive difficulties would be easy to identify by such routine procedures as a program intake interview. This is not always the case. Many subtle but important disruptions in cognitive functioning may not be obvious to a casual observer. Many factors, such as a good vocabulary, prior educational achievement, an assertive personality, and a history of successful vocational performance, may mask declining mental abilities. Furthermore, many people who experience a gradual decline in brain function may be unaware of their difficulties, even when they gradually become quite an impairing factor in daily life. They may not understand the nature of their concerns or may perceive their increasing difficulties in life functioning as a function of bad luck, uncooperative coworkers, antagonistic family members, and other external factors. They may seek to remedy decreased vocational performance by seeking additional and more specialized training and education. Even when the nature of cognitive difficulties becomes clear to them, some clients will adopt an attitude of denial, minimizing the deficits they experience, and attempting to stabilize their vocational performance by working extra hours, taking work home, or double- and triple-checking their work products.

This discussion of neuropsychological functioning in MS rehabilitation has three goals. These include:

1. Developing an awareness of what the major cognitive concerns in MS rehabilitation are and how to assess those concerns;
2. Developing an understanding of the implications of cognitive status difficulties as they relate to job functioning; and
3. The development of applied skills using a case study model.

A major area of misunderstanding in the assessment of cognitive functioning is the equating of intellectual status with overall cognitive status. Briefly, the concept of intellectual functioning focuses on a relatively narrow band of overall cognitive functioning. Clinically, intellectual functioning is defined by performance on standardized intelligence tests. Unfortunately, intelligence testing is highly influenced by factors such as level of education, level of social sophistication, and a number of "static" abilities, such as knowledge about a culture and past experience. When working with populations that may have cognitive dysfunction, reliance on limited factor measures such as intelligence tests may completely miss glaring problems. Because of the way in which intelligence tests are constructed, these tests may sometimes reflect a better picture of past performance or capacity than of present potential.

Neuropsychological testing involves the nonmedical identification and measurement of brain-based abilities. As contrasted with testing for intellectual status, neuropsychological testing reviews many different aspects of brain functioning. Also in contrast to IQ testing, neuropsychological testing has a greater focus on adaptive abilities as opposed to static abilities: it is less sensitive to past learning and more sensitive to a person's ability to presently adapt to an environment. Although it may seem paradoxical, many people with CNS disease who have high tested IQs (i.e., 120 or higher) may still have pervasive deficits in neuropsychological functioning, even to the point where they are rendered unemployable. Another distinction between neuropsychological tests and tests of intellectual functioning is that neuropsychological tests are designed specifically to distinguish people with impairment in brain functioning from people with normal brain functioning. Table I-6 in Section I reviews several areas important to adaptive functioning that can be measured by neuropsychological testing.

Neuropsychological Concepts Important in Vocational Rehabilitation

The following narrative reviews the concepts presented in Table I-6. It should be noted that these functions are somewhat arbitrarily defined, and there may be some overlap between them. They are, however, presented as a convenient way of conceptualizing functions that are important in vocational rehabilitation.

Sensorimotor Integrity

Sensorimotor integrity is perhaps the most basic area reviewed by neuropsychological batteries. Multiple sclerosis may involve lesions that affect motor control and strength. It may also blunt or alter normal sensation, to a greater or lesser degree, depending upon the location and number of lesions. Sometimes MS will generate sensation, such as the pain involved in Lhermitte's condition. While neuropsychological testing may not pinpoint the exact site at which lesions are causing this disruption, it is desirable to document and quantify these concerns (see Table II-1). Neuropsychological assessment generally attempts to provide indices in the following areas: fine motor control in the fingers and hands, the ability to distinguish subtle tactile sensations presented simultaneously, the ability to distinguish subtle sounds presented simultaneously, and a gross examination of peripheral vision and field of vision. A neuropsychological examination ordinarily does not include a review of gait, balance, and sensory function in areas other than the hands and face. The neuropsychological evaluation also includes tests for dysarthria (problems with speech function related to sensorimotor impairment involving the muscles used to form speech sounds).

TABLE II-1   Sensorimotor Integrity

- Do the areas of the brain responsible for controlling the body's muscles function efficiently?
- Does the brain efficiently process input from sensory organs?

Implications of Decreased Sensorimotor Ability (depending upon portion of the brain affected by MS)

- Decreased fine motor abilities
- Difficulty with gait and ambulation
- Possible paralysis
- Dysarthria
  — Decreased communication
  — Psychological impact

Vocational Implications

As regards dysarthria and communicative abilities, sensorimotor function has far-reaching implications in the vocational arena. Dysarthria involves slowness in motor speech and indistinct and garbled wording, and often creates a psychological barrier as well as inefficiency in verbal communication. The social and psychological impacts of dysarthria may have significant effects, on both the client and coworkers.

Other vocational implications of decreasing sensorimotor function will vary greatly according to the occupation considered, with obvious implications for the trades or occupations requiring dexterity and speech, and in potentially physically dangerous working environments. Vocational interventions in this area may include a host of assistive technology strategies including orthopedic appliances; assistive equipment to help with fingering, manipulating, or hand-guiding material; electric wheelchairs; voice-activated computer systems; optical and electronic devices for magnifying images; and so forth. People with adequate neuropsychological functioning in other areas may still experience considerable difficulty with sensorimotor deficits. As with the specific example of dysarthria, social and emotional (e.g., self-esteem) barriers can be created that may hamper the effectiveness of an otherwise well-qualified individual.

Attention and Concentration

Attention may be defined as the ability to focus on a given stimulus. Concentration is the ability to maintain that focus, both over time and in the presence of distractors. The realm of attention and concentration may be considered a "gateway" concept, as performance in other areas of functioning is likely to be degraded by problems with attention and concentration (see Table II-2).

TABLE II-2   Attention/Concentration
■ Attentive—The ability to attend to individual stimuli ■ Concentration—The ability to focus attention on a stimulus in the presence of distractions or for an extended period of time **Vocational Considerations for Attention/Concentration** ■ Minimize sources of distraction ■ Minimize disrupting interpersonal contacts ■ Resimplify or reorganize work tasks ■ Review variables such as anxiety, physical fatigue, pain, and depression

Vocational Implications

The basic qualities of attention and concentration make them defining parameters in many occupational situations, and otherwise capable individuals with significant problems in this area will experience the greatest difficulty in performing many types of work. Interventions for people with difficulty in attention and concentration may involve a number of physical modifications to the job site such as locating a work site in an area relatively free of distracting elements, minimizing interpersonal contact, less busy work shifts (e.g., late afternoon or early evening), erecting cubicles or noise buffers, and so forth. In some situations the use of a timer, a checklist of work tasks with "completion deadlines," or electronic reminder signals may be helpful in keeping a client on task or remembering key elements of a job sequence. Simplifying work tasks or reorganizing them into a different format may also be useful interventions, depending on the specific nature of the job. Variables such as anxiety, physical fatigue, pain, and depression frequently interfere with an individual's attention and concentration. For people who already experience difficulties in this area, the aforementioned variables may compound the problem.

Memory Function

Memory may be conceptualized in a variety of ways (see Table II-3).

TABLE II-3   Memory

- Visual-spatial
- Verbal
- Long-term
- Short-term—Generally more problematic than long-term
- Incidental or random

Vocational Considerations for Memory

- "Low-tech" memory aids
  - Memory books, tape recordings, PDAs
  - Calendars, including electronic
  - Self-reminders
  - Watch alarms
- "High-tech" memory aids
  - Computerized reminder or paging systems
  - Computerized memory books

For most people with MS, remote memory (i.e., memory for personal history, events in the past, and past learning) remains intact. When difficulties with memory function occur, they are more likely to involve short-term memory, memory for recently learned information and incidental memory, or memory for information not specifically focused upon. An example of incidental memory would be remembering, at a later time, the color of a suit worn by a person to whom one is introduced casually.

Memory can also be logically divided into memory for verbal material and memory for visual or visual-spatial material. These two aspects of memory appear to be served by different cortical locations, and one may have a significant decrement in one of these areas with the presence of adequate performance in the other. The consistency with which one remembers random facts is critical to successful life performance. Memory is, as suggested above, an ability highly dependent on concentration and attention. Neuropsychological tests for memory attempt to assess short-term memory for both visual and spatial abilities and to some extent incidental memory. Some tests for memory also involve procedures that allow the practitioner to infer how much a testee may benefit from a situation in which memory cues are utilized or rehearsed.

Vocational Implications

As with attention and concentration, the vocational implications of memory are enormous, and in many ways memory also serves as a "gateway" concept with respect to other functions. Otherwise capable individuals with significant memory dysfunction are likely to have the greatest of difficulty in any but the simplest and most routine of tasks. In the assessment of memory for vocational purposes, it is especially useful to ascertain the degree to which memory function improves with practice or repetition. Some practitioners will routinely include tests to assess this function, such as the California Verbal Learning Test, Selective Reminding, or the Rey Auditory Verbal Learning Test, which assess this benefit within a framework of random facts to be remembered. It may be desirable to specifically request from a practitioner testing to assess this function of memory. In many jobs (e.g., that of an expeditor or manager), one needs to be able to "retain random facts." Verbal memory measures with the "paragraph context only" will miss assessing this capacity for storing random information items.

Vocational interventions for memory are many and varied. Their usefulness to a given individual will also vary. One of the most successful "all-around" memory interventions is the training of an individual to use memory books, paper and electronic appointment calendars, computer templates, checklists, written self-reminders, watch alarms, and other "low-tech" approaches. When people are willing and able to implement use of these devices, much improvement can be made with decreased memory function. A variety of high-tech computer and memory book type of interventions of varying degrees of complexity are also available.

Language Abilities

Neuropsychological evaluation of language ability is focused on the assessment of language as a communication device as opposed to more superficial factors such as vocabulary or spelling. Included in this definition are written language, spoken language, and other forms of symbolic communication such as arithmetic (see Table II-4). Language abilities can be viewed in terms of expressive language, or the ability for communication, and receptive language, or the ability to understand language input. The expressive–receptive paradigm applies to both written and spoken language as well as to symbol systems such as mathematics (see Table II-5). The term *aphasia* is used to describe impairment in language function, and neuropsychological testing investigates the possibility of both expressive and receptive aphasia. Cognitively based difficulty with language, or aphasia, is distinguished from difficulty with motor speech or dysarthria, as reviewed in the section on sensorimotor integrity.

In addition to possible problems with expressive and receptive language, two other language-based concerns appear as difficulties with overall brain function increase. The first of these is difficulty with complex language. As the overall efficiency of an individual's brain decreases, it may become increasingly difficult to expediently process and comprehend language that conveys a lot of information (see Table

TABLE II-4   Definitions of Language Ability and
Expressive and Receptive Language

Language Ability:

The ability to understand language and to use language to express ideas

Expressive Language:

The ability to communicate language output to others

Receptive Language:

The ability to understand language input

TABLE II-5   Definitions of Expressive and Receptive Aphasia

Expressive Aphasia:

Difficulty generating understandable language

Receptive Aphasia:

Difficulty understanding language input

II-6). Accordingly, an individual may have increasing difficulty with sentences that convey more than one piece of information or with conversations that shift rapidly from one topic to another. A second language-related concern is that of abstract language. Many people with increasing difficulty in brain function suffer a reduction in the ability to abstract, as discussed in the appropriate section below. People who have difficulty with abstraction often have difficulty with simile, metaphor, acronyms, and other figures of speech. The aphorism "a golden hammer breaks down an iron door," may be seen as a statement of the prevalence of virtue over baseness by an individual with no difficulty in abstraction. It may be uninterpretable or interpreted only in a narrow and literal manner by a person with increasing difficulty in the ability to use symbolic language.

Vocational Implications

A breakdown in language functioning, and the attendant breakdown in communication with one's interpersonal environment can have the

TABLE II-6   Language-Based Concerns and Vocational Considerations

Language-Based Concerns for People with Decreased Brain Function

- Complex language (too much information or too much structure)
- Abstract language (simile, metaphor, acronyms, figures of speech)

Vocational Considerations

- Simplify language output

greatest implication for vocational performance. In addition to the obvious problems with supervision, learning a job task, and interacting with co-workers, a breakdown in language abilities frequently has counseling implications with respect to anger, frustration, depression, and similar concerns. Language-related abilities are generally thought to be centered in the left temporal lobe in most individuals.

Visual-Spatial Ability

The concept of visual-spatial abilities refers to a host of nonverbal abilities generally involved with visual-spatial and perceptual motor abilities (see Table II-7). These include the ability to deal with two- and three-dimensional formats, perceive whole-to-part relationships, and perceive field–background relationships. These generally are considered to be right temporal or right temporal parietal lobe abilities and may include aspects of nonverbal problem solving and reasoning.

Vocational Implications

People with difficulty in visual-spatial abilities may have a number of concerns that will directly affect employment. These may include alterations in depth perception, difficulty coordinating the hands or the feet with visual input, difficulty distinguishing field from background, problems with estimation of distance and size, and similar concerns. Difficulties in visual-spatial abilities may also have some effect on problem solving and abstractional ability.

TABLE II-7   Visual-Spatial Ability

The ability to deal with two- and three-dimensional formats, perceive whole-to-part relationships, perceive field–background relationships

Cognitive Flexibility

Cognitive flexibility refers to the ability of a person to deal efficiently with simultaneous stimuli or to move quickly from one stimulus or situation to another. A person with decreased cognitive efficiency tends to have difficulty doing multiple tasks or switching between several complex procedures (see Table II-8).

Vocational Implications

In the modern workforce, more and more jobs emphasize a high level of cognitive efficiency. Even jobs with modest pay ranges, such as those in the fast-food industry, ask for a good deal of cognitive efficiency. This ability, or *multitasking* as it is called in the workforce, is essential in obtaining more responsible jobs. People with intact intellectual abilities who suffer decrements in cognitive efficiency are frequently in the frustrating position of being limited to employment options considerably below their intellectual potential. This ability thus serves as a "gateway" affecting the capacity to express other vocational abilities in the workplace. It is difficult to offer effective remediation for problems with cognitive inefficiency in the workplace. To some extent, an attempt to organize the workplace efficiently, or to make use of assistive technology, as described under the section on memory and in other text sections, can be helpful. Organizing the work flow to minimize the necessity to perform tasks "simultaneously" or in quick succession may be useful. The more complex (and well

---

TABLE II-8   Cognitive Flexibility

- The ability to efficiently perform simultaneous tasks or tasks in the presence of distractors
- The ability to screen out extraneous stimuli
- Multitasking
- Highly important in the modern workforce
- Gateway concept that puts upper limits on use of other abilities in a vocational context.

---

paying) a job becomes, the more unique and challenging are these interventions.

Executive Functioning

Problem solving and abstractional ability represent the highest order of cognitive functioning (see Table II-9). These are termed executive abilities and involve a spectrum of brain-related abilities, including organizing, initiating, sequencing, abstraction, problem solving, the ability to benefit from environmental feedback, and self-monitoring. Executive functioning is thought to be mediated by the frontal lobes, as damage to the frontal lobes frequently causes decrements in executive functioning. People with increasing difficulty in executive functioning may begin to have difficulty understanding the nature and degree of their concerns. In more extreme cases, this may result in their being unaware of or discounting difficulties with behavior or performance that seem obvious to other persons (see Table II-10).

Vocational Implications

As difficulties with brain function increase, problems with executive functioning set a limit on possible job complexity and responsibility.

TABLE II-9   Highlights of Executive Functioning and Behavioral Concerns

---

Executive Functioning

- Abstraction
- Problem solving
- Self-regulation
- Initiative
- Motivation

Behavioral Concerns

- Lack of awareness
- Denial of disability
- Decreased social judgment

TABLE II-10   Executive Functioning
As with cognitive flexibility, executive functioning serves as a "gateway" that sets upper limits on expression of other vocational abilities in the workplace

As with cognitive efficiency, efforts to simplify the workplace or organize and restructure the workload may be helpful in dealing with some abstractional ability difficulties. Teaching self-management skills with respect to developing strategies for reviewing work, comparing work to established paradigms or self-evaluation checklists, and working within a timeframe can be useful. At the extreme end of the spectrum, decreased executive functioning (e.g., lack of motivation, inability to self-regulate) may preclude competitive employment. In cases of more moderate involvement (e.g., poor problem solving skills and some impaired judgment), increasingly close supervision and higher levels of structure will be helpful (see Section III on the benefits of job coaching or a paid coworker as mentor).

Patterns of Neuropsychological Deficit in Multiple Sclerosis

Much recent work (e.g., Rao, 1991, 1995) has suggested that people with MS, as a population, may evidence specific patterns of neuropsychological impairment. While neuropsychological impairment in MS is, in theory, correlated with lesion location and lesion load, a statistical review of cognitive difficulties, as measured by neuropsychological batteries, suggests a tendency for difficulties in three areas (see Table II-11).

Care should be taken in making prior assumptions about a patient's neuropsychological status without the benefit of neuropsychological testing. Nevertheless, difficulties in these areas may be the first cognitive signs of impairment due to MS lesions. Because many patients will attempt to accommodate difficulties in cognitive functioning in many ways (e.g., spending extra time on tasks to ensure optimal performance, denial, or avoidance of problematic situations),

TABLE II-11   Patterns of Neuropsychological Impairment in Multiple Sclerosis

- Decreased short-term memory/attention
- Decreased cognitive efficiency/speed of processing
- Decreased executive functioning (i.e., problem solving, abstraction, decision-making abilities)

(Rao, 1991; 1995)

the use of standardized neuropsychological testing is often the best strategy to assess cognitive functioning.

Initial difficulties with short-term memory seen in patients with MS appear to be more related to retrieval of learned information rather than an inability to form a memory, as patients frequently perform more adequately on tests involving cueing than on tests requiring unaided recall. This is a useful finding, as it suggests the utility of memory strategies such as reviewing and transcribing recently learned information. Many individuals experiencing memory difficulties begin to adopt such strategies as note taking and additional reliance on schedule books and electronic calendars or calendar notes. The use of rehearsal or transcribing strategies represents another step in memory strategies, and patients may need specific training in this skill.

Difficulties with memory function, cognitive efficiency, speed of information processing, and reduced executive functioning may become first apparent in their effect on a patient's vocational status, as these are areas of function that will have direct implications for productivity.

Neuropsychological Batteries

The two most commonly used neuropsychological batteries in the United States are the Halstead–Reitan Battery (Reitan & Wolfson, 1985) and the Luria–Nebraska Battery (Golden et al., 1984) (see Table II-12). The Halstead–Reitan Battery represents the approach most frequently used in the Northwest/Western United States and will be the example reviewed in depth in this volume. The Halstead–Reitan

TABLE II-12　Commonly Used Neuropsychological Batteries
Halstead–Reitan Battery (Reitan and Wolfson, 1985) Luria–Nebraska Battery (Golden, 1984)

Battery is a so-called *fixed battery*. Fixed batteries are those that routinely use a standard set of test measures on each new testee. They feature tests that are well normed and are applied in the same manner to each individual. This is in opposition to the so-called *flexible battery* strategy in which different measures may be chosen for different testees, depending on the presenting complaint and the hypothesis of the neuropsychologist. Fixed batteries have the utility of allowing comparison from one patient to another, are especially useful in a research context (because they offer a more quantifiable patient profile), and allow a vocational rehabilitation practitioner to better develop an experiential base in neurologically oriented rehabilitation planning.

Obtaining a Neuropsychological Evaluation

A point has been made that, when making inferences about discrete brain function, only neuropsychological tests, as opposed to tests for general intellectual functioning or aptitudes, are appropriate measures. A neuropsychological test is rarely administered in the absence of other test input (e.g., measures of emotional and intellectual status). In some research situations, information from neuropsychological tests alone is sufficient for the purpose. In applied situations, however, such as vocational programs, neuropsychological tests are generally administered by a neuropsychologist in combination with tests of intellectual function and emotional status. In practice, the term *neuropsychological evaluation* generally refers to the administration of a neuropsychological battery, augmented by tests of intellectual status such as the Wechsler Adult Intelligence Scale-III, and by tests of emotional or psychological status, such as the Minnesota Multiphasic Personality Inventory I or II (see Table II-13). The reason for this is that in many practical situations in neuropsychological

TABLE II-13   Neuropsychological Evaluation

- Neuropsychological tests
- Tests of intellectual functioning (i.e., Wechsler Adult Intelligence Scale)
- Tests of emotional or psychological status (i.e., Minnesota Multiphasic Personality Inventory)

vocational rehabilitation (i.e., vocational counseling, life care planning, or assessment of residual ability) a person's spectrum of functional capacity is most likely to be a function of three variables: intellectual, emotional, and neuropsychological status.

Working with the Neuropsychologist

Choosing a Neuropsychologist

There is no nationwide certification or licensing procedure for psychologists. Each of the 50 states has its own licensing criteria for psychologists, and none licenses psychological specialties such as clinical psychology, counseling psychology, or neuropsychology. Rather, practitioners take a single licensing examination and practice in fields dictated by their training, professional experience, and developed interests. Although bound by professional ethical standards to practice only within areas of competency, no specific legal statutes apply, and psychologists are expected to be self-governing in this area. While this practice allows for flexibility and the application of knowledge and skills gained "in the field," it calls for thorough screening of a potential neuropsychological consultant.

How, then, can those who advertise as "neuropsychologists" have their training and background evaluated? It is helpful first to understand what training options are available to psychologists who wish to specialize in neuropsychology. Before contracting for neuropsychological services, a useful screening strategy is to request the resumé or curriculum vita of a potential practitioner. People offering neuropsychological testing services for vocational purposes should be able to demonstrate academic and field experience that establish their competency (see Table II-14). Credentials can include specific pre- and postgraduate training in neuropsychological test administration, scoring, and interpretation. A supervised postdoctoral internship in neuropsychological practice should be included. American Psychological Association (APA) approved training sites and programs attempt some measure of consistency and thoroughness of training and can be an indication that a practitioner has received adequate training in the area. A specialty board certification administered through the American Board of Professional Psychology/American Board of Neuropsychology offers an advanced credential termed a *diplomate*. Achieving diplomate status involves meeting adequate ABPP/ABCN academic and training criteria, as well as peer review of work samples and an oral examination by other neuropsychologists of diplomate status. Although a psychologist not otherwise qualified might achieve a degree of competency in neuropsychology through informal means, such as independent reading, attending workshops, and participating in training strategies, none of these strategies is likely to offer the comprehensive and intensive training available in formally designed neuropsychology programs. Because there is currently no universal agreement on the training and experience that qualifies one to practice as a neuropsychologist, the preceding guidelines may aid in choosing a competent practitioner for vocational rehabilitation purposes.

Referral Questions for Neuropsychologists

The identification of a qualified neuropsychologist is important in providing neuropsychological assessment services for vocational reha-

---

TABLE II-14   Choosing a Neuropsychologist

- Obtain resumé or CV
- Graduate training in neuropsychology
- Supervised doctoral internships in neuropsychology
- American Psychological Association (APA) accreditation
- Diplomate status in neuropsychology

---

bilitation. Even within the pool of people qualified to offer neuropsychological services, however, there may be great variability in an individual practitioner's ability to translate test results into vocationally useful information. Many good diagnosticians may have relatively little experience in relating neuropsychological test results to vocational concerns. The concern of the vocational rehabilitation professional is not a good diagnosis per se, but the translation of test results into vocationally relevant or functional statements. To further this end, carefully written referral letters, accompanied by detailed job descriptions (even task analyses) whenever possible, are an indispensable tool.

Following is a list of suggested questions and areas to be explored by a neuropsychologist (Table II-15). Although the list is not exhaustive, it is exemplary of the types of questions and the ways of phrasing questions that may be most useful in ensuring that useful test data become a relevant part of the vocational evaluation. It is important to keep in mind that most neuropsychologists will have considerably less direct vocational or rehabilitation experience than will the referring rehabilitation professional. It therefore is not desirable to ask questions that assume specialized vocational knowledge on the part of the neuropsychologist. Accordingly, questions such as "Can Sally be expected to perform well in retail sales?" may place unrealistic expectations on

---

TABLE II-15   Referral Questions for Neuropsychologists

- Operationally framed questions
- Do not assume vocational expertise on the part of the neuropsychologist
- Include curriculum or course descriptions of proposed training (if applicable)
- Identify assets as well as deficits
- Ask for discussion of remediation of deficits
- Solicit help on communication strategies
- Include job description or ideally task analysis of new job or work return goal
- Ask questions about client fatigue, persistency, ability to self-correct, and consistency of performance over the course of a day

---

the practitioner's ability to respond adequately. Framing questions operationally is one manner of addressing this concern. A more useful way of framing the question about retail sales would be a series of operational questions: "Can Sally be expected to perform well in a situation that involves ongoing, but cursory social interactions with 25 to 65 people from the general public within the course of a day? Can she be expected to learn and retain data, such as pricing structures and product lines, that may change on a weekly basis? Will she be able to efficiently attend to customer needs in the presence of other distracting elements such as noise in the workplace, interruptions from supervisors and coworkers, and ambiguous requests from customers?" Again, the benefit of a specific job description on a function/task level or the actual opportunity to visit the work site is often very helpful.

The following are some specific points of inquiry that may be helpful in guiding the neuropsychologist to produce vocationally useful reports.

1. Ask for an identification of specific client assets as well as deficits and problem areas. Some clinicians are simply more "problem-oriented," have been trained that way, and will spend more time discussing potential deficits than potential assets. In an applied situation, such as vocational rehabilitation, the identification of assets is as important as is the identification of deficits. Some neuropsychological deficits or problems may not be functionally relevant.

2. When reviewing areas of deficit, ask for a discussion of how these may be accommodated or remediated. It is especially helpful to ask what type of social or physical environments will most readily accommodate areas of neuropsychological weakness. An example of this would be the restructuring of the workplace to provide an area of relative quiet and freedom from distraction for a person who has difficulties with divided attention and concentration.

3. It is useful to solicit help from a neuropsychologist on communication strategies. Even for people with relatively intact language abilities, deficits in other areas such as concentra-

tion, abstraction, and memory can indirectly impair communication ability. Because language abilities tend to be over-rehearsed skills, variables such as a well-developed vocabulary or good listening and attending skills may mask basic difficulties with language usage. A specific review of communicative abilities is essential to adequate vocational rehabilitation planning.

It can be very useful to include medical and psychological records in a referral for neuropsychological services. The presentation of adequate medical and psychological data may aid the neuropsychologist in making decisions about otherwise equivocal results. As a general rule, the availability of medical and/or psychological data will make a neuropsychological diagnosis more accurate and provide the practitioner with a context within which to frame assessment results.

4. If a specific vocational training goal is in mind at the time of referral, the inclusion of the curriculum or course descriptions can be an asset in framing the questions asked of a neuropsychologist. As discussed previously, the most useful means of framing training or later related job descriptions are in operational terms that do not presuppose specific occupational knowledge on the part of the practitioner—neuropsychologists often complain about being asked to provide vocational recommendations in a vacuum of actual job understanding.

5. It can be useful to ask questions about client fatigue, persistence, the ability to self-correct, and consistency over the course of a day. In neuropsychological testing, an attempt is made to get clients to perform at maximum ability. It can be useful, especially in vocational situations, to ascertain the ability of a client to persist on a task throughout the day and to explore what may be the impact of fatigue, motivation, distractibility, and other variables.

If one expects to request services on a regular basis from a neuropsychological practitioner, it can be advantageous for the rehabilitation professional to pay for a direct neuropsychological feedback session. Most practitioners will be willing to provide this service, and the additional expenditure of funds (i.e., up to one hour of a psychologist's time on each report) may be useful in developing a knowledge and expertise base for the rehabilitationist, while helping to shape the neuropsychological practitioner's future responses in a more vocationally relevant manner.

Case Study: Sample Neuropsychological Evaluation

Referral Information

Date of Evaluation: December 12, 2047

Ms. Jane Smith is a 47-year-old, right-handed female referred for neuropsychological evaluation by the Division of Vocational Rehabilitation. Ms. Smith has been employed as a junior high school teacher by the Fontana School District in Fontana, Nebraska, for the past 17 years. She presents with two-year-old-complaints of decreasing memory efficiency, fatigue, and feeling "swamped."

Ms. Smith's medical history is negative for loss of consciousness, electrical shock, infectious disease with fever, anoxia, or seizures. Ms. Smith earned a bachelor's degree in special education and completed one year's graduate study at the University of California–Bakersfield (UCB), subsequently becoming employed by the Fontana School District. She indicated no difficulties with cognitive functioning until the present. Medical history is positive for MS, diagnosed four months before her referral to this center.

Tests Administered

The following instruments were administered: the Halstead–Reitan Neuropsychological Battery, the Wechsler Adult Intelligence Scale-III (WAIS-III), the Wide Range Achievement Test-IV (WRAT-IV), the Stroop Test, the Seashore Tonal Memory and Rhythm Test, the WAIS-III Figural Memory and Verbal Memory Test, the California

Auditory Verbal Learning Test (CAVLT), the Controlled Oral Word Association Test (COWAT), Reitan's Aphasia Screening Test, a sensorimotor screening inventory, and the Wonderlic Personnel Test, Form B. Emotional status was reviewed via the Minnesota Mulitphasic Personality Inventory-II (MMPI-II).

Observations

Ms. Smith was alert and cooperative during the 5.5 hours of this examination. She verbalized concerns and self-doubts during portions of the WAIS Memory Test and on the COWAT, although she appeared well motivated to complete all measures. During one test of problem-solving ability on the Halstead–Reitan Battery, she teared briefly after several failures but continued to task completion.

Test Results/Interpretation

Intellectual functioning was assessed using the WAIS-III. A Full Scale IQ of 115, with a Verbal IQ of 119 and Performance IQ of 110 were observed. These scores fall at the 84th, 90th, and 75th percentiles when compared with the appropriate age norms. Some difficulty was observed on the Performance subtest Digit-Symbol, which involves a multitasking procedure in which the numbers between 0 and 9 are matched with arbitrary codes. In general, performance-related scores tended to be in the average range, with scores on verbal subtests falling between the high average and superior ranges.

Of 16 tests of neuropsychological functioning (an expanded Halstead–Reitan fixed battery), 10 (62%) were performed outside normal limits. The greatest single trend was a tendency for short-term memory measures, both verbal and visual-spatial, to be performed slightly outside the normal limits. Indices of attention and concentration were performed inconsistently, with some measures performed adequately and others outside the accepted performance limits. Although performance in this area did not vary greatly from the established norms, there is evidence for at least a mild dysfunction of attentional and concentration abilities. Academic testing generally was within the range expected for the observed IQ, although performance on tests of standard arithmetic was somewhat lower than might have been expected. No concerns with aphasia were noted and no dysarthria was noted. Instruments measuring problem solving and abstractional ability were performed adequately. Some mild difficulty in performing a task of alternating attention was observed. The sensoriperceptural examination was performed normally. Some motor slowing was observed bimanually on the finger oscillation test. Strength of grip was somewhat weaker bimanually than would have been expected.

Turning to the assessment of emotional status, a valid profile was obtained on the MMPI-II. Significant elevations were observed on four scales. People with similar profiles are frequently described as anxious, tense, and reactive. There may be a focus on somatic complaints, and the possibility of converting psychological concerns to physical complaints is indicated. The likelihood of at least a moderate degree of depression is indicated.

Summary

This is a 47-year-old female with MS, presently employed as a junior high school teacher. Neuropsychological testing suggests a mild degree of cognitive disruption with mild to moderate difficulty in tasks involving attention, concentration, and memory. There is some motor slowing bimanually and a modest decrement in strength of grip bimanually vis à vis established norms.

Intellectual functioning was found to fall in the average to high average range, with verbal measures performed somewhat more adequately than performance measures. Academic testing is generally within the range suggested by her education and IQ. There may be some modest difficulties with cognitive efficiency.

Strengths include intact language, high average IQ scores, and adequate problem solving and abstractional abilities. Testing suggests some disruption in psychological functioning, with an MMPI-II profile indicating at least a moderate degree of tension and anxiety. A somatic focus is indicated, with the possibility that this patient may convert psychological symptoms into physical symptoms. A moderate level of depression may be present.

This patient is not seen as "disabled" from the standpoint of her present employment, although these results suggest that she may be experiencing some inefficiency in carrying out her duties. The extent to which psychological distress interferes with her cognitive functioning is not known, although there may be an interactive effect in this area that should be explored.

Questions of Interest: Potential Recommendations

Discussion: Actual Report Recommendations

1. It is likely that this patient will perform more adequately in employment situations that are relatively well structured and minimize elements of distraction and interference with her primary task.

2. The job description reviewed in connection with this evaluation suggests that there is a high level of multitasking involved in Ms. Smith's present position. Attempts to minimize this factor, such as the use of a teacher's aide, may be useful in increasing Ms. Smith's performance. A mixed, less arduous class load, with study hall monitor responsibilities, etc., may prove helpful.

3. Because MS generally is a chronic and a progressive condition, it may be desirable to involve Ms. Smith in developing a long-term plan for utilizing her skills and abilities within the school system in a situation that is less demanding than classroom teaching. Although she is seen as appropriately placed in the classroom with modest accommodations, contingency planning should begin early.

4. The provision of supportive psychotherapy is strongly recommended. Supportive psychotherapy does not imply the presence of innate psychopathology, but rather is a standard rehabilitation recommendation when a plurality of environ-

mental stressors may temporarily overwhelm an individual's adaptive resources.

5. The neuropsychological deficits reviewed herein are in the mild to borderline range of impairment. It is not possible to determine the extent to which psychological concerns (i.e., reactive depression, increased somatic concerns) contribute to the overall picture. It may be desirable to readminister tests which fell outside normal limits in a year's time.

6. An important goal of the supportive therapy recommended above should be the review of Ms. Smith's depressive concerns, which are assumed to be reactive to her current difficulties with MS. Should these not alleviate, consideration of more aggressive psychotherapy and/or consideration for a trial on antidepressant medication should be weighed. A program of modulated exercise might be considered.

7. Ms. Smith might also benefit from being assigned a teacher mentor or mentoring coworker (even from another school) to assist with work organization, perhaps prioritization, coping strategies, and maybe lend some emotional support.

Please feel free to call me if you have additional questions concerning this patient.

Summary

This section reviewed the importance of neuropsychological evaluation in vocational rehabilitation. The point was made that a relatively high number of people with MS will experience significant difficulty with cognitive functioning. This suggests that some review of cognitive status should be a more routine, rather than an incidental, procedure in MS vocational rehabilitation unless an individual obviously is functioning quite adequately. A screening that better assesses areas in which those with MS often have neuropsychological deficits can be helpful and efficient from a cost perspective.

The importance of neuropsychological testing as a tool in cognitive evaluation was stressed. Neuropsychological testing, which tends to stress adaptive ability, was identified as the preferred means of reviewing cognitive status. Other inferences of cognitive status, such as measures of intellectual functioning, measures of vocational aptitude, and review of scholastic or vocational achievement may have the dual disadvantage of lacking a broad-based overview and of relying on historical, rather than current adaptive ability.

Some suggestions with respect to working with a neuropsychologist were offered. These included the utility of framing questions in an operational manner, of providing detailed referral letters outlining specific areas of concern, and of providing the neuropsychologist with referring data such as medical charts, job descriptions or analyses, course load demands, and similar information.

References

Arnett, P.A., Rao, S.M., Grafman, J., Bernardin, L., Luchetta, T., Binder, J.R., and Lobeck, L. (1997). Executive functions in multiple sclerosis: An analysis of temporal ordering, semantic encoding, and planning abilities. *Neuropsychology* 11(4):535–544.

Brassington, J.C., and Marsh, N.V. (1998). Neuropsychological aspects of multiple sclerosis. *Neuropsychol Rev* 8(2).

Golden, C.J. (1984). Applications of the standardized Luria–Nebraska Neuropsychological Battery to rehabilitation planning. In P.E. Logue and J.M. Schear (eds.), *Clinical neuropsychology: A multidisciplinary approach*. Springfield, IL: C.C. Thomas.

Grafman, J., Rao, S., Bernardin, L., and Leo, G.J. (1991). Automatic memory processes in patients with multiple sclerosis. *Arch Neurol* 48(1):1072–1075.

Rao, S.M. (1995). Neuropsychology of multiple sclerosis. *Curr Opin Neurol* 8(3): 216–220.

Rao, S.M. Leo, G.J., Bernardin, L., and Unverzagt, F. (1991). Cognitive dysfunction in multiple sclerosis. I. Frequency, patterns, and prediction. *Neurology* 41(5): 685–691.

Reitan, R.M., and Wolfson, D. (1995). *The Halstead–Reitan Neuropsychological Test Battery: Theory and clinical interpretation*. Tucson, AZ: Neuropsychology Press.

Vocational Rehabilitation Intervention

Robert T. Fraser, Ph.D., C.R.C.

Multiple sclerosis (MS) is one of the more complex disabilities to be encountered from a vocational rehabilitation perspective. LaRocca (1995) summarizes the scope of the problem (see Table III-1). He indicates that more than 90 percent of individuals with MS have worked and more than 60 percent were working when diagnosed. This, in fact, represents higher occupational functioning than that of the general population. People with the disability often are well educated and often appear to encounter disability onset and its associated impairments in mid-career. If the disease progresses, LaRocca (1995) indicates that employment often drops away, with only 20 to 30 percent of the population working 10 to 15 years from diagnosis.

Although a variety of symptoms are involved and impact vocational functionality, major issues include impaired mobility and motor function, fatigue, cognitive concerns as discussed, mood fluctuations, bladder problems, vision concerns, and a chronic progressive course, which can interact with age at diagnosis (a poor prognosis with older age) and educational level (the lower the level, the worse the prognosis). There has appeared a longstanding tendency, as noted by LaRocca, for women to drop out of the workforce in greater numbers than men. In coping with this complex illness, it can be difficult enough for a woman (often a primary home manager) to focus on

---

TABLE III-1   What Is the Employment Picture for Adults with MS?

- 90% have a work history
- 60% working at time of diagnosis
- 20–30% working at 10–15 years from diagnosis
- Majority of population is women with post-secondary education

---

(LaRocca, 1995)

housekeeping and child care alone—she generally is unable to maintain the additional vocational role given the disability's complications. In these cases, the husband becomes the principal financial earner, and the wife with the MS disability often tends to secure Social Security Disability Income (SSDI) support and/or disability pension.

Findings from the more recent Project Alliance effort (NMSS, 1997) suggest that fatigue and cognitive impairments appear to be common and significant barriers to effectively performing in the workplace (see Table III-2). Other issues such as visual impairment, spasticity, difficulties with fine motor functioning, heat sensitivity, and emotional issues were lesser concerns than these two major work-related barriers. On a positive note, Verdier-Taillefer and coworkers (1985) indicate that certain environmental variables can ease the burden of working, such as public sector employment, jobs that were sedentary in nature, and work sites in which accommodations could be easily made. Public sector job may be more accommodating.

Project Alliance determined through survey efforts that employers thought certain accommodations (e.g., flexible scheduling, physical modifications to a work site, or adaptive equipment) were generally reasonable (see Table III-3). It is of interest, however, that for those individuals with more severe disabilities, the accommodations that would be most helpful (e.g., rest periods or flex shifts, home-based

---

TABLE III-2   Project Alliance Findings: Major Barriers to Employment

---

- Fatigue
- Cognitive impairments

(NMSS, 1997)

TABLE III-3   Project Alliance Findings

■ Employers feel that certain accommodations are reasonable (e.g., flexible scheduling, work site physical modifications, or adaptive equipment)

■ Employers resist most helpful accommodations (e.g., rest periods, home-based work, or a support person at work)

---

employment, or a support person at work), were generally considered unreasonable to employers. At the time of Project Alliance, employers believed that the latter types of accommodation would send a negative message to other coworkers. These attitudes, however, may be changing with the number of individuals conducting work from home increasing dramatically and the blatant need for skilled employees, given the almost full employment in the U.S. economy as we began the millennium.

The current labor market may be an ideal arena for new, targeted, proactive vocational rehabilitation efforts for and on the part of individuals with MS. New inroads might now be made relative to flexible work scheduling, home-based employment, or different models of employment support (e.g., paid coworker as trainer and support person). When there is a distinct need for manpower in the workforce, an employer may be more receptive to "accommodation" in all its diverse forms.

A Brief History of MS Vocational Rehabilitation

LaRocca (1995) emphasizes that there has been relatively minimal focus on vocational rehabilitation efforts in MS rehabilitation. Over the years a number of different demonstration projects have been attempted, which were recently reviewed by Rumrill and coworkers (1996) (see Table III-4). These projects included the MS Back to Work or Operation Job Match (1980), the Job Raising Program (1993), the Return to Work Program (1983), the Career Possibilities Project (1994), and the multisite Project Alliance (1997). The projects were funded chiefly by the Rehabilitation Services Administration through

TABLE III-4   MS Employment Demonstration Projects

- MS Back to Work or Operation Job Match (1980)
- Job Raising Program (1983)
- Return to Work Program (1993)
- Career Possibilities Program (1994)
- Project Alliance (1997)

a mixture of efforts by individual MS chapters, universities, and more recently the National Multiple Sclerosis Society (NMSS) (see Table III-5). The initial projects in this sequence of efforts involved helping people through job-seeking skills training and providing job placement assistance with an MS-specific job bank or employer mentoring effort. Later projects maintained the job skills training component but put an increasing emphasis on empowerment strategies, placement planning, and strategizing solutions for job site barrier removal. There is no question that later projects, specifically Project Alliance (NMSS, 1997), were influenced by the implementation of the Americans with Disabilities Act (ADA) of 1990.

The focus of the most recently completed Project Alliance was to coach the project participant with MS to take a more proactive employment site stance (Table III-6), the idea of early intervention with the employer and the "still employed" participant with MS being optimal. The rehabilitationist met with the employer and employee with MS to encourage open discussion and strategize job accommodations to maintain job stability before termination or resignation occurred. This more recent vocational rehabilitation approach encour-

TABLE III-5   Evolving Nature of MS Specialized Projects

- **Early programs**—Job seeking skills emphasis, group context with direct placement assistance, or employer mentor
- **Later programs**—Maintain job seeking skills
  - Empowerment emphasis, group context, return to work/ accommodation strategizing

(Rumrill et al., 1996)

TABLE III-6   Multi-site Project Alliance Components

- Early intervention with employer and employee—open discussion of issues
- Job site analysis
- Report formulation with accommodation recommendations
- Follow-up as to retention

(NMSS, 1997)

ages early accommodation and empowering client accommodation self-efficacy—teaching the client to maintain his or her job. The earlier projects, therefore, focused on job seeking skills teaching, group support, and placement assistance while later projects moved more toward a self-empowerment, accommodation skill teaching, or employment negotiation model.

Certainly, a number of these efforts are exemplary, with the combination of job-seeking skills training, job development, and even direct community employer support being very positive. The earlier projects were relatively successful, but they had more difficulties assisting clients who had already established Social Security subsidy support, specifically SSDI. The latter projects, in their emphasis on early intervention, self-accommodation strategies, and self-empowerment, began to rely less on specific job development efforts (see Table III-6). Of those who were able to fully participate in Project Alliance to include full job analysis of their activities, 85 percent were still working at follow-up. Unfortunately, only about one-third of the program participants engaged in the project to the point of a complete job analysis (see Table III-7). Open communication with the employer can

TABLE III-7   Project Alliance Findings

- Cautiousness of clients to let the VR specialist meet the employer (one-third followed through)
- People with this disability don't often seek vocational help
- Of the third fully engaging in Project, 85% employed at follow-up

(NMSS, 1997)

be blatantly neglected; opening up to a full range of job site intervention may be perceived as "too risky" by the employee with MS.

On an overview, the projects, to date, seem to highlight the following needs (see Table III-8):

1. The importance of an individualized approach for these clients due to the complex nature of the disability and its physical complements, but also the frequency of residual cognitive concerns. An individual vocational assessment option should be available within any type of program in MS vocational rehabilitation, including neuropsychological screening. Potential cognitive concerns need to be considered as part of the vocational assessment process.
2. Clarification of an individual's financial support needs, within the context of one's disability severity, is critical. Some clients, as an example, will need to maintain their SSDI and can only earn up to $740 on a part-time basis (as of 2/01). Other individuals may be able to earn more by utilizing a Social Security Plan for Achieving Self Support (PASS) or a plan for Independent Work-Related Expenses (IWRE) (e.g., to pay for adaptive equipment). In any case, the projected financial status needs to be reviewed because it will affect vocational goal setting and plan implementation.
3. Client accommodation self-effectiveness and self-advocacy with an employer is important whenever possible (see Table III-9). This involves knowledge of one's individual accom-

---

TABLE III-8   MS Vocational Rehabilitation Projects, To Date

Highlight:
- Importance of individualized vocational assessment, including neuropsychological status
- Clarification of financial/subsidy issues
- Importance of effective accommodation strategizing
- Need for a range of effective job placement models, including home-based

---

TABLE III-9   Accommodation Self-Effectiveness

An individual with MS:
- Knows accommodation needs
- Understands accommodation under ADA
- Is encouraged to approach employer
- Role plays, following a model, an accommodation presentation

---

modation needs, an understanding of the ADA, and comfort in approaching an employer to specifically present these needs (having prepared through scripting, role play, video presentation, etc.). Agency rehabilitation staff can be used to perform job analysis, and provide input on accommodation funding support, tax incentives, and related information. Successful accommodation can be key to job retention, with early intervention being optimal.

4. It is important to underscore that different placement approaches will need to be used in dealing with the multiplicity of issues as presented by the MS disability. A "one size fits all" type of vocational rehabilitation placement approach simply is not adequate and does not reflect an optimal vocational rehabilitation approach. The need for selective or "niche" placements, often in part-time work, must be considered.

5. Because fatigue is such a critical issue and travel often is physically draining, *a home-based work option should be considered for a number of individuals with MS* (employers are likely to accept home-based work part of the time).

LaRocca (1995) references the fact that the NMSS did not really engage the employment challenge until the early 1990s. In 1991, the Society prepared a position paper on employment. The paper emphasized the following points:

- Disability by itself should not be assumed to reduce one's employability.
- The Society would take a lead role in implementing the ADA.

- Work site accessibility is a critical issue.
- Small accommodations can make a significant difference relative to work adjustment and job maintenance.
- It is a critical societal responsibility to change the negative attitudes regarding the employability of individuals with disabilities.
- The reduction of current work disincentives legislation is imperative to providing truly viable employment options for those with severe disabilities.
- There is a continuing need for legislation that provides employer incentives to hiring those with disabilities.
- The federal–state vocational rehabilitation (VR) system needs modification to allow it to better serve individuals with MS.
- There is continuing need for research to better understand employment concerns, issues resolution, and better uses of technology.
- There is a need for a national comprehensive long-term care system for those with the disability.
- The NMSS strongly supports organizations with affirmative action plans for people with disabilities.
- Programs and policies for those with disabilities should reflect input from service consumers with the disability.

This was truly a bold step forward for the national society. Less than 50 percent of the National MS Society affiliates nationally were even addressing employment concerns as part of their intake process at that time. Furthermore, the majority of chapters had only partial contact with employers and state vocational rehabilitation agencies. Agreements between societies and state VR agencies had never resulted in improved vocational rehabilitation services for clients with MS. The contacts that were made tended to be with specific individual counselors, who were perceived as invested in the MS cause, for purposes of service provision.

Policies and Program Perspectives

Rumrill (1996) continues to emphasize referrals for clients with MS to state vocational rehabilitation services, the development of early intervention strategies focused on self-advocacy and accommodation to help people with MS keep their jobs, and ongoing employment assistance. He underscores that every work-motivated client with MS is an appropriate referral for vocational rehabilitation services. If an individual wants to work or needs some assistance in maintaining a position, referral must take place. Rumrill (1996) endorses earlier findings by Rubin and Roessler (1995), in which research findings linked successful rehabilitation factors such as client motivation and residual abilities versus disability severity to successful rehabilitation. In order for many individuals with MS to maintain momentum, they will need support not only from vocational rehabilitation staff or a job-seeking skills group, but also from family members, significant others, their peers, and other allied health care providers. Those who leave the workforce (e.g., women, older workers, and those with higher family incomes) often do so voluntarily (Rumrill, 1996) and not always for the right reasons—vocational rehabilitation consultation and community support might result in a different decision-making process or outcome.

Vocational Assessment

Roessler (1996) emphasizes that the initial emphasis should be feasibility assessment of *returning to the same job or a related job* as quickly as possible, particularly if a client enjoyed the work. Diverse computer software can be used for this purpose—programs such as OASYS (published by Vertek, Bellevue, WA) can actually identify companies within one's county or city with related jobs. Often whether a person can return to a prior or related position within a company relates to *financial or accommodation issues* that can be negotiated.

   For many individuals undergoing a vocational evaluation to identify new job possibilities within their present company or within a community at large, certain elements of the vocational evaluation are very specific. Certainly, many components of the traditional areas assessed such as vocational interests, intellectual abilities, aptitude and academic achievement patterns, personality propensities, work values, etc. can be very important; but there are a number of concerns presented by the population with MS that require some "fine-tuning" in order for the vocational rehabilitation effort to be a success. Areas of clarification include the following (see Table III-10):

- An understanding of the unique number of issues relating to MS such as a client's type and severity of disability, potential issues with spasticity, motor coordination concerns, possible tremor issues, physical weakness, bladder function, visual impairments, dysarthria, dysphasia, or even sexual dysfunction concerns—which are common, typically for men. Neurologists or often a neurologist–psychiatrist team can be in the best position to evaluate these concerns and plan treatment interventions. There are other tools that can be helpful in terms of better understanding this disability. The Expanded Disability Status Scale (EDSS), developed by Kurtzke (1981) can be valuable in quantifying disability's impact—the scale scores traditionally have been associated with vocational rehabilitation outcome. This relationship should probably be discounted because vocational outcome will be better with a more detailed vocational assessment and tailored placement accommodation intervention effort. Gulick (1986) also has an MS Activities for Daily Living Self-Care Scale, which measures 15 critical items related to an individual's community functioning

TABLE III-10   Vocational Assessment: MS Particular Concerns

- Understanding unique physical aspects of disability
- Financial status/subsidies
- Cognitive strengths and weaknesses
- Emotional status—Depression and anxiety
- Rehabilitation outlook
- Type and availability of social support
- Needed accommodation—The Work Experience Survey

and psychosocial adaptation. The Personal Capacities Questionnaire (PCQ) and the Functional Activities Inventory (FAI) by Crewe and Athelston (1984) are other tools helpful in clarifying an individual's capacity for independent and optimal psychosocial living. An individual with MS and his or her significant other or family members can often be most helpful in providing more accurate or complementary information related to the scales.

■ The financial picture—Within the context of the severity and extent of their MS-related impairments, many individuals may not be able to attempt full-time work and may need to focus on part-time work. As of this book's publication, it is possible for individuals on Social Security Disability Income to earn up to $740 monthly without loss of Social Security subsidy. Some individuals, in consideration of the severity of their impairments and the monthly cost of their medications (e.g., $1,300) can simply not afford to lose Social Security subsidy and medical treatment support. These financial concerns need to be "hammered out" early in the vocational rehabilitation process (see Table III-11).

For those on SSDI, the costs of a computer, automobile, assistive equipment, etc. might be deducted from earned income as an IWRE. If not, a technology that is helpful to working might be deductible as a medical expense. A person might need to establish a nine-month period of work trial while their earnings are not counted as income until the final ninth month and they have proven their work capabilities.

TABLE III-11   Work Access Financial Considerations

■ PASS plan
■ IWRE
■ Medical expense deductions
■ Job trial
■ AmeriCorps stipend
■ Other options

Some individuals can work as AmeriCorp volunteers, a VISTA-like program through which a stipend of approximately $800 a month can be received that does not count as income. Individuals on Supplementary Security Income (SSI) can utilize a Plan for Achieving Self-Support (PASS) to lower income due to work-related expenses and maintain Supplemental Security Income (SSI) payments. Mendelsohn (1996) reviews some of these concerns in more detail, but *work access or return can require some pragmatic financial thinking* given each individual's subsidy structure.

The Ticket to Work and Work Incentives Act of 1999 also remediated two major work return disincentives. Those receiving Social Security who return to work will receive premium free Medicare coverage for 4.5 years beyond the current limit. Additionally, effective January 2000, former Social Security beneficiaries losing their jobs due to their established medical condition may have Social Security income subsidy immediately reinstated while their situation is being evaluated—this reinstatement request must be made, however, within five years of Social Security's or Supplemental Security's income termination.

■ Cognitive pattern—For clients with MS seeking vocational rehabilitation services, cognitive concerns are prevalent. These issues are reviewed in more complete fashion in Section II. Consequently, they are not discussed in great detail here. It should be noted, however, that for many years these issues often were blatantly overlooked by both client and service providers in the rehabilitation process. The Project Alliance final report (1997) highlighted some of these cognitive concerns within the MS vocational rehabilitation literature for the first time. Dr. Clemmons proposes an economic battery for identifying some of the common attention, concentration, cognitive flexibility, and memory issues that can be in evidence. It should be noted that the new WAIS-III, as an IQ test, will identify some of these concerns more clearly than the earlier WAIS measures. When testing of this nature is not possible, for whatever reason, a community-based assessment or job tryout should be used when there is a suspicion of cognitive deficits. It is much better that these issues are clarified when they do exist and compensatory strategies implemented before these cognitive issues bring about a competitive job loss or marginal performance.

- Emotional concerns—Minden and Schiffler (1990) suggest that there is a range of emotional difficulties impacting individuals with a diagnosis of MS. These include depression, anxiety, emotional lability, euphoria, and so on, with depression being particularly salient. In general, there should be some probing in the clinical vocational interview relative to anxiety or depressive symptomology. In some cases, additional psychometric instruments should be used such as the Center for Epidemiological Studies' Depression or Anxiety Scales, the state section of the State-Trait Anxiety Inventory, or the MMPI -II, through which depression and anxiety can be identified, as well as other types of DSM-IV Axis I or II concerns.

  Some individuals, particularly the newly diagnosed, will simply profit from some time to adjust. They will benefit from educational groups and other types of available support that allow them to make continuing progress relative to life functioning or, at a minimum, psychosocially stabilize. Other individuals will require psychotherapy including cognitive behavioral, insight-oriented, and stress management or inoculation training. Some of the group will benefit from an antidepressant or other pharmacotherapy approach, often in tandem with psychotherapy. These concerns and interventions are discussed in more detail in Section IV. Nonetheless, this area deserves attention. *There will often be no substantive vocational rehabilitation progress unless these emotional issues are identified and managed as necessary.*

- Rehabilitation outlook—In Roessler's 1996 article on assessment, he highlights use of the Goldberg Scale (1992), which gauges an individual with MS's rehabilitation outlook (e.g., back to work motivation, realistic assessment of capacities and limitations, and optimism about future recovery and rehabilitation after treatment). Roessler endorses use of the scale, believing that the client's self-perspective or sense of optimism plays at least as important a role in vocational rehabilitation success as the severity of the disability. It is our observation that some of this rehabilitation outlook can also begin to change as a function of a targeted vocational support group or a job club involvement. With training in accommodation strategies, handling of benefit issues, and so forth, a client's self-confidence and motivation can increase. Much of this is basically the easing of job-related uncertainty. Individuals who are uncomfortable with receiving federal or other subsidies often remain specifically motivated for work return. Clients' perception of their vocational and social support systems can also be part of this rehabilitation outlook. In a current vocational rehabilitation demonstration project involving those with MS at our Center, we are currently using the HOPE scale by Herth (1992) as a means of measuring this "rehabilitation outlook" or sense of optimism, and then later relating it to actual placement outcome.

- Available social support—The construct of social support is very important. Due to the multiple human systems that can be compromised for the individual with MS, it remains important as part of the vocational rehabilitation assessment "package" to review the type and level of social support that is available. Some of the available social support scales are somewhat complex. The scale we utilize simply examines who is available to provide emotional, personal appraisal, general information, and needed physical support (including transportation) for each client (client self-report) (see Table III-12). It also asks the client's satisfaction with the type of support that is available within each of these support categories. It can be of interest to review client and significant other or caregiver incongruencies relative to the perception of who is available for support in each area.

TABLE III-12   Social Support Questionnaire

1. Who accepts you totally, including both your best and worst points? Who provides you with emotional support?

   Names:_____

   _____

   _____

   Overall satisfaction with support

1	2	3	4	5	6
very dissatisfied					very satisfied

2. Whom can you really count on to tell you in a thoughtful way, when you need to improve in some way or to give you personal feedback about how you're coming across?

   Names:_____

   _____

   _____

   Overall satisfaction with support

1	2	3	4	5	6
very dissatisfied					very satisfied

3. Whom can you count on to give you important information about work, home life, money, and finance issues?

   Names:_____

   _____

   _____

   Overall satisfaction with support

1	2	3	4	5	6
very dissatisfied					very satisfied

4. Whom can you count on to help you out and do things for and with you when you really need them?

   Names:_____

   _____

   _____

   Overall satisfaction with support

1	2	3	4	5	6
very dissatisfied					very satisfied

■ Reasonable accommodation and assistive technology assessment—Recent Project Alliance findings underscore that fatigue and cognitive concerns are the primary barriers encountered by those with MS (see Table III-13). Roessler and Rumrill (1995) indicate that among the cognitive concerns, key issues relate to remembering (48%), speaking (46%), working under stress (42%), and thought processing or speed of information processing (44%). Physical concerns related more to writing (48%), handling (45%), heat in the workplace (38%), adequate vision (34%), walking (30%), and other lesser concerns (see Table III-14).

A job analysis can be very helpful, but the Work Experience Survey (WES) by Roessler and Gottcent (1994) walks the client through the identification of specific accessibility barriers, the essential functions of the job, job mastery concerns, job satisfaction issues, and finally works toward clear barrier identification with an emphasis on recommending the client's own solutions or who might be able to help. When one reaches the final stage of barrier and solution generation (section six of the survey), it is helpful to brainstorm under three categories: job procedural solutions, physical modifications to the work site, or the use of assistive technology (tending to be equipment) (see Table III-15). If pressed for time, completion of this later section and three and four of the WES are critical to solution generation.

Many of the accommodations in MS rehabilitation are likely to be procedural due to a combination of both cognitive

---

TABLE III-13   Cognitive Concerns

- Memory—48%
- Speaking/Communicating—46%
- Thought processing—44%
- Performance under stress—42%
- Judgment —16%

(Roessler and Rumrill, Jr., 1995)

TABLE III-14   Physical Concerns

- Writing—48%
- Handling—45%
- Heat in the workplace—38%
- Walking—30%
- Considerable standing—28%
- Working 8 hours—28%
- Work pace—24%

---

problems and physical fatigue (see Table III-16). Physical modifications to a work site tend to be rather basic: allowing physical ease of access or work site positioning closer to an entrance or closer to the bathroom. Assistive equipment tends to be relatively low cost and involves memory book aids, personal digital assistants (PDA), palm top computers, air conditioners (combating heat effects), larger computer screens, and voice-activated software. Electronic aids for purposes of remembering or organization have become particularly common in our society and can be easily purchased and recommended by occupational therapists, speech and language pathologists, or consulting assistive technologists or assistive technology clinic teams.

- One of the greatest benefits of referral to a state vocational rehabilitation agency can be the funding of an assistive technologist who can assist the client with MS to find solutions to barriers pinpointed through use of the Work Experience Survey (WES). Again, for most individuals with MS, common accommodations are going to be procedural, particular-

---

TABLE III-15   Categories of Job Accommodation

- Procedural change
- Work site modification
- Use of an assistive device
- Involve several of the above

TABLE III-16   MS Rehabilitation Procedural Accommodations

- Decreased workday
- Flex time arrangements
- Restructure job
- Some task reassignment to co-worker
- Job sharing
- Telecommuting
- Job coach/coworker as trainer
- Provision of some physical assistance

ly flex time and reduced hour workdays. For additional accommodation information of all types, the reader is referred to the Job Accommodation Network (JAN) at West Virginia University (phone 800-342-55260) or web site: www.csuchico.edu/abilcon/DR/gen/janbbs.html or ABLE-DATE in Newington, Connecticut (203-667-5405) or web site: www.abledata.com.

Why the Intermediate Level of Assessment?

At the end of the first or basic level of the vocational assessment process, it is critical that specific recommendations be provided relative to vocational reentry or job access directions. In relation to vocational reentry, the critical question is whether an individual can return to the same job with or without specific accommodations. As discussed previously, these accommodations can be procedural, involve some type of physical changes to the work site, or the use of assistive equipment. In other cases, new job goals are established and it becomes apparent that an individual can enter a new occupation with some supportive brokerage by rehabilitation staff to employers within the community. Other individuals will need some type of tailored approach (e.g., a job share) or a specific type of employment support (e.g., a job coach or paid coworker as trainer). An option in the procedural category of accommodation is flexible work that is home-based. Based on initial assessment data, the desired route to competitive work is often quite clear. In other cases, *particularly due to complex physical or overt or subtle cognitive issues,* the suggested route to competitive placement (or whether this effort is even feasible), remains very unclear. It then becomes critical to use an intermediate level of community-based assessment for further information and direction. The next section therefore reviews this intermediate level of assessment.

The Intermediate Level of Assessment: Community-Based Job Tryouts

Due to the complex nature of issues affecting adults with MS, it often is difficult to make a prognosis about the effectiveness of a specific approach to vocational stabilization. This becomes even more difficult when one needs to consider the range of potential accommodations available through the ADA. It is often the case that mid-career adults need to have accommodation considerations for a job in which they were formerly proficient and now may be unsure about their capabilities—the previously discussed Project Alliance showed the benefits of early intervention focused on optimal job accommodation strategies.

Fortunately, in 1993, the U.S. Department of Labor established a national job wages waiver based on pilot project findings in the state of Washington (see Table III-17). The waiver allows individuals with disabilities to *work within the private sector on an unpaid basis* for purposes of *vocational exploration, assessment, or training.* From a formal perspective, the waiver allows 5 hours of vocational exploration, 90 hours of vocational assessment, and 120 hours for actual vocational training (see Appendix A). There are, of course, a number of waiver requirements related to a worker not displacing other workers or pro-

TABLE III-17   Department of Labor Non-Paid Work Experience Waiver

5	hrs for vocational exploration
90	hrs for vocational assessment
120	hrs for vocational exploration
Total	215	hrs per specific job tryout

viding a company with a competitive edge over others. A tremendous benefit for the individual with MS is that this "job tryout" block of hours can be broken down in any fashion (e.g., 15 hours per week or split shifts) to start the work reentry effort. It enables clients to practice "in vivo" accommodation techniques to discern whether they can perform on a prior job or a new job.

During this intermediate level of unpaid assessment, workers compensation insurance specific to the job being tried is provided by a monitoring state vocational rehabilitation agency or one of their vendors. A tremendous benefit to this approach is the collection of data helping to identify the type of placement model that might be needed given specific physical, sensory, or cognitive concerns. In some cases, it can be determined that an individual may need a coworker mentor (e.g., an architect) to problem-solve certain issues (e.g., architectural plan segments) over lunchtime, after work, before the beginning of the workday, and so on. The best arrangement is for these coworkers not to simply volunteer, but to be compensated for their work through a formal arrangement at their hourly salary level. For individuals with certain physical limitations (e.g., balance), certain work segments might be traded with another worker who could handle an occasional climbing concern, as an example. In some instances, it can be reasonable to pay a coworker or a member of the community to provide *physical assists* on a periodic basis. A standard protocol is usually utilized to track trainees' productivity, accuracy, various job and interpersonal behaviors, and so forth while they "try out" under this waiver; job performance can be gauged with and without accommodation.

It should also be noted that individuals can work within nonprofits as volunteers (e.g., within a medical center) if viable jobs exist for purposes of tryout—insurance coverage is then provided by the non-profit as it is for other volunteers. It should be noted that if a client with MS is *residing* within a medical or rehabilitation facility, volunteer work status is legally contraindicated. They need to be paid for their services on a commensurate level to other workers or after being "selectively certified" in accord with Department of Labor regulations for a lower wage based on their reduced productivity as related to an "average worker" in a specific job class.

Choice of a Placement Approach

Following review of input from the basic vocational assessment, integrating available neuropsychological information and often the intermediate, community-based type of evaluation, an approach to placement must be chosen. In each case, the client's physical status, financial status, interpersonal functioning, the workplace demands and available support from supervisor or coworker must be considered. As reviewed in Section II, subtle cognitive or neuropsychological issues are going to be common, often approximating up to a 60 percent range within a rehabilitation population. Potential issues in the cognitive arena will often need to be considered. For some individuals, therefore, data from both the preliminary vocational assessment and a later community-based job tryout must be carefully reviewed. Figure III-1 is a model from earlier work in traumatic brain injury revised more specifically to the needs of the population with MS.

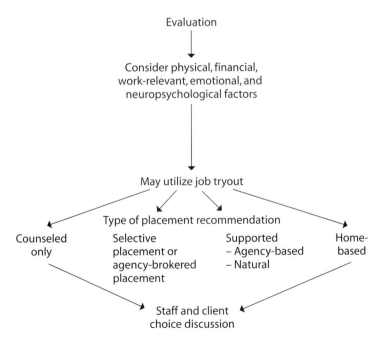

FIGURE III-1   Placement model decision tree in MS rehabilitation.

Participant choice, it must be noted, is still a very active component of this model despite vocational rehabilitation counselor, job coach, or rehabilitation team perspective. A compromise can often be reached if opinion differences exist, with a job tryout or community-based assessment being used to establish capacities or clarify misperceptions of ability. In some cases, the placement approach decision can be somewhat arbitrary (e.g., a decision between a job coach or coworker support is easily supported by the client's preference). Some clients, often those with cognitive deficits, sometimes will want no supports at the job site—if this cannot be endorsed by staff, the client may "go it on their own" with some advisement and/or perhaps return for a support model if a failure occurs. Differences in choice of a placement approach between VR staff and program participants with this disability do not, however, frequently occur.

A succinct discussion of each model follows below:

- Vocational counseling and advisement *only*—Based on preliminary vocational evaluation findings, many clients are quite capable of organizing their own job searches. They may profit from rehabilitation staff advisement, job leads for informational interviews, community contacts, or feedback on their accommodation strategies; but they definitely do not need to be brokered to employers by a vocational rehabilitation specialist. Clients with more severe MS will often need practice or actual tutelage in presenting their accommodation needs and solutions from a physical perspective alone. For many individuals, improving their job search or interview strategies is truly empowering to job getting and keeping. This is not to say, however, that in addition to counselor support, these individuals would not benefit from involvement in a vocational group or job club format. In addition to improving job search techniques, emotional support from a group can improve both self-esteem and confidence while lowering levels of anxiety and depression.

- Selective placement or direct brokerage by a rehabilitation agency—In this case, because of a client's involved physical limitations or additional cognitive impairments, accommodation considerations and financial negotiations with an employer can become quite complex. It can be critical that a rehabilitation counselor, placement specialist, or job coach be directly involved in brokering a client to the employer and assisting in negotiating viable accommodations. The NMSS (1997, p. 18) has indicated that a majority of employers want to spend less than $1,000 on accommodations and almost two-thirds were concerned about accommodations and cost. Additionally, more than 50 percent of the employers were concerned about absences, the ability of an individual with MS to maintain a hectic work pace, fluctuations in the individual's capacity related to the disability, a person's inability to perform as efficiently on the job as previously because of the condition, and so forth (NMSS, 1997, p. 19). The employer often will look to the rehabilitation counselor, placement specialist, or job coach as a credible reference or endorser of a client's capacities, in addition to their role of providing input relative to accommodation strategies. This is often the key reason that a client is brokered to an employer by an agency, in addition to the need for more expedient placement or work access.

Reasonable accommodation for many individuals with MS will not involve assistive equipment, but more often procedural changes (e.g., a split schedule or flex time, a rest period, telecommuting or home-based employment options, etc.) and some work site modification (e.g., work site closer to a bathroom, conveniently arranged equipment or supplies, etc.). For some companies, procedural changes in how a job is done are actually more threatening than the use of assistive equipment or conducting physical modifications at the work site. Again, the rehabilitation counselor or placement specialist can be a key person in negotiating these accommodations, especially procedural, while reassuring the employer of a job candidate's merits as an employee. Clients with MS, particularly those with cognitive issues, are often not going to be able to navigate and resolve these issues alone.

■ Agency-provided job site support—A number of different types of supported employment approaches have been used within the United States (see Table III-18). These include small business types of supported employment programs with a mixed workforce of individuals with and without disabilities, a mobile work crew with one or more supervising job coaches, and an "enclave" within the private sector in which individuals are coached until they can reach the productivity levels of those without disabilities in similar types of company work activity. Due to the complex level of professional positions held by many mid-career professionals experiencing the onset of MS, the *traditional job coach model* will often not be appropriate. *It will be helpful only in a minority of cases.*

This is principally because the vast majority of clients (chiefly women) have post–high school education and were not working in the unskilled work sector or even within the lower end of the semiskilled work sector. The job coach model, however, would still be very applicable for those needing assistance when entering an unskilled or semiskilled position. Wehman and coworkers (2000) have described this model in detail as applicable to individuals who in general have more severe neuropsychological impairment. A variant of the Wehman model involves agency support involving payment to a "consultant" (e.g., community college welding instructor, retired pharmacist, accountant, etc.) who mentors

TABLE III-18   Agency-Provided Supports

■ Supported employment models
  — Enclave
  — Small business-entrepreneurial
  — Mobile work crew
■ One-to-one job coach
■ Community "job consultant"
■ Physical assistant

an individual on an as-needed basis to the point of consistent job task proficiency. These types of mentors or job coaches are really advising within a professional or upper-end semi-skilled level of work activity. Some of these individuals are members of retired professional associations and will do the activity as a volunteer. The benefit to these types of consultants is that they can make themselves available on weekends or evenings and do not intrude directly on the job site. A concern, however, is whether they are able to assist the person with MS directly on tasks and work products that relate directly to the client's actual work setting.

Some types of job site support as provided by an agency are directly physical in nature (e.g., transportation to work, assistance in toileting, etc.). A physical assistant may initially be provided by an agency, but often will eventually become a paid employee of the worker with MS. The cost of this type of physical assistive support may be paid under a Social Security Plan for Achieving Self-Support (PASS) or the IWRE mechanism, which reduces net income and results in Social Security financial subsidy levels not being affected.

- Natural supports in the workplace—The use of natural supports in the workplace has been reviewed in the rehabilitation literature by Storey and Certo (1996). Coworkers and job site supervisors often can be helpful to an individual with a disability in the workplace on an informal or formal basis (see Table III-19). State divisions of vocational rehabilitation personnel have been writing on-the-job training (OJT) agreements for clients for decades. These have usually been successful training programs, subsidized by a state agency (e.g., client's salary paid to the company at 50%) over a several month period of training. Curl and coworkers (1996) have formalized a procedure in more directly using paid coworkers as trainers. Curl and colleagues have completed more than a decade of research utilizing this model. The core of the model is a training sequence that involves describing a task to a trainee, showing a task, observing the individual

TABLE III-19	Natural Supports in the Workplace

- State VR on-the-job training agreement with the supervisor or coworker as trainer
- Direct coworker as trainer model

(Curl et al., 1996)

performing the task, and providing feedback in relation to proficiency. Additionally, training tools for both the trainer and the trainee are outlined as needed based on the specific issues encountered. Curl and colleagues provide a formal training manual and accompanying videos relative to the procedure (Curl et al., 1987, a, b, c, 1990).

A paid tutorial session involving a four-hour block of training (which can be done in sections) is usually conducted for new coworkers in order that they understand the approach and the different tools that they can use to improve workers' accuracy or productivity on the job. Trainer tools can involve the specific set-up of the work area, the use of a one-minute reminder, using bonus and warning notices, basic task checklists, timers, self-evaluation checklists, etc. The approach deals not only with job proficiency, but also with interpersonal and other job-related behaviors. The article by Curl and coworkers (1996) reviews utilization of this model as it applies to individuals with traumatic brain injury returning to semiskilled or skilled levels of work activity.

In consideration of the general educational skill levels of most individuals with mid-career onset MS, this paid coworker as trainer approach appears to be highly applicable. Generally, a job coach hired by a rehabilitation agency, often having a degree in psychology or education, will simply not have the skill base to coach an electronic technologist, a nurse, an attorney, architect, etc. This can only be done by a skilled coworker or "peer" who will meet with the individual at specific times or intervals (lunchtime, on break, etc.) on a daily or as-needed basis until the trainee for a new job or returning employee with MS is more consistently effective and efficient in his or her daily work. This approach for individuals with a prior base of job experience in the recent project by Curl and associates (1996) appears to be relatively inexpensive. In this particular project, the amount of mentoring funds paid to coworkers averaged only $400 at 17 months (Fraser et al., 1997). Many individuals doing complex work activity may need only occasional mentoring or prompts from a coworker, but these can occur at certain critical times during a day or week and are important to getting the job done competently. It often is untenable to maintain job coaches at a work site for these isolated critical instances, even if they were able to understand the complexity of the specific work activity. The paid coworker can meet this "on the spot" mentoring need, even for professionals, at costs that seem to reduce quite dramatically within weeks.

- The home-based work option—In the United States home-based employment and telecommuting dramatically increased during the 1990s (see Table III-20). Telecommuting will be a substantive part of workforce activity in future years. Some estimates are that 40 percent of today's workers will be telecommuting at least part-time within the next few years (Rumrill et al., 2000).

  For many years, home-based work activity was considered an anathema in rehabilitation circles. The thinking toward this type of activity was that it was not occupationally or socially "mainstream" and was limited to basic assembly

---

TABLE III-20   Home-Based Employment for the Client With MS

- Telecommuting an available "mainstream" work option
- Reduces physical and cognitive fatigue for the client with MS
- Can provide some flex time options as needed
- Fits with the professional, often computer literate, skill level of the population with MS

tasks, envelope stuffing, and so on. Due to the advent of the computer, the "virtual workforce" is now able to maintain online company contact and perform computer-based work activities in addition to telephone and transmission activities all from one's home. For the person with MS, particularly during periods of disability exacerbations, home-based activity can truly be the most practical. Some individuals are able to work until they reach a maximum fatigue level, then rest, and again resume work activity as they are physically energized. Individuals might also work based on their critical cycles of energy and mental alertness (e.g., mid-afternoon to early evening) or avoid the heat of the day when this is an issue. On a very basic level, home-based work reduces commute time, which is both physically and cognitively fatiguing for many individuals (with this disability), or in other cases simply mitigates basic physical or health risk concerns. As so much of today's work activity is based on Internet commerce or other computer-based communication, now is an ideal time to consider job development for clients who truly need the home-based option.

In many cases, state vocational rehabilitation can pay for computers and other assistive equipment. Social Security PASS or IWRE plans can be used to reduce income while enabling an individual to secure equipment critical to carrying out the telecommuting work activity. In general, companies are open to this model because home-based employment lowers real estate rental, parking space costs, and other logistical costs of doing business. Additionally, the home work option tends to reduce employee turnover and, therefore, employer recruitment and training costs. Home-based employment often results in increased productivity and less employee downtime during the workday. Telecommuting can also increase responsiveness to customers because home-based employees (particularly beneficial for many with MS) can vary their workday (e.g., work evenings) and make access to a company representative much easier for the consumer.

Telecommuters can also live at some significant distance from a company, sometimes out of state, which results in improved company geographical coverage and lower phone costs.

■ Blended forms of support—It might be noted that in order to effect a successful placement, specifically in MS rehabilitation, it may be optimal to utilize several types of support models in effecting a successful vocational rehabilitation. For example, an individual with MS might work at home on a split shift in order to decrease fatigue. While in training, the company may receive on-the-job training funds to reduce the cost of a client's training time or learning curve. Additionally, a paid coworker might visit the client at home on a weekend, on lunch hour, etc. in order to provide helpful mentoring or tutelage. The more vocational impairments experienced by an individual, the greater blending of placement models might occur in effecting a successful rehabilitation outcome (e.g., part work at home and part work at a company). In order to achieve successful vocational rehabilitation, staff are only hampered by their lack of creativity. "Thinking outside the box" is encouraged and might best be considered a norm in MS vocational rehabilitation (see Table III-21). A client on SSDI might work part-time, from 3 to 7 P.M., and earn less than $740 a month for Social Security purposes due to an IWRE plan utilized for assistive equipment. Additionally, this individual could be tutored part-time by a retired professional paid by the rehabilitation agency while also receiving mentoring from a paid coworker who visits the home work site to provide mentorship relative to specific company procedures.

TABLE III-21   Case Example: Client with MS and Cognitive Issues Returns to Work

■ Receiving SSDI of $1,200 per month
■ Earning <$740 on a 3–7 pm job
■ Paid coworker mentors on the job
■ Retired volunteer does some at-home tutoring

Case Study: Rehabilitation Planning in MS Rehabilitation

The Case of Jason

To encourage "brainstorming," we now review the case of Jason and discuss this case from two perspectives; first, identifying any additional information that is needed for purposes of appropriate evaluation and specific goal setting. Second, once this information is fully complete, you will be asked to respond to rehabilitation placement plan questions. The specific intake information on Jason is provided below:

- Psychosocial History—Jason is a 28-year-old man who grew up within a professional family with both his siblings being quite socioeconomically successful. He is a law school graduate and a former university tennis star. The onset of MS occurred six years ago. He encountered increasing symptoms during his last year of law school. He could not pass the bar exam post-graduation given several attempts and has no substantial job experience. He does some part-time legal consultative work for his father's real estate business on a monthly, contractual paid basis. As opposed to support from "competitive" work, this appears to be his father's effort to provide ongoing financial support. The contractual arrangement, however, will soon end with his father's retirement from his real estate partnership. Jason is unsure of a vocational direction.

- Medical Status—Jason has been treated with methylprednisone twice in the last year in a small Minnesota town. His MS had shown a chronic progressive course but has stabilized to slightly improved over the last six months. He has difficulty with fluctuating visual disturbance and motor coordination when walking. He is not particularly limited by distance and does not require a cane, but he does have a wide and mildly ataxic gait. There also is some slowing of dexterity in his finger manipulations. He is being treated with dibenzyline and amantadine, respectively, to improve coordination and reduce fatigue.

- Cognitive Functioning—Jason presents himself as an accomplished writer. In fact, he had some short stories published several years ago. He also displays and is very proud of his legal dissertation. He appears articulate and has a strong vocabulary. There is no testing as to his current cognitive abilities available.
- Emotional Functioning—Jason appears to have fluctuating difficulties with anxiety and depression. He has trouble returning to sleep after awakening to urinate during the night. Dating has been limited despite returning to the northwest several years ago and presenting as an attractive male. He is also limited socially by his finances, but he attempts to maintain contact with former fraternity brothers and college social contacts within the area.

Questions and Preliminary Planning

Before we can begin active vocational rehabilitation intervention with Jason, there is more information that a vocational rehabilitation counselor might need for purposes of assessment and in planning specific interventions that might be implemented as you continue in vocational goal setting activities (see Table III-22). Please take time to review and consider the services and preliminary interventions that might be needed across the following categories:

TABLE III-22   What Assessment Information
Would Still be Helpful in Jason's Case?

- Medical
- Other allied health team assessments/Consultations
- Psychological/Neuropsychological
- Psychiatric
- Vocational
- Other?

Case of Jason: Questions of Interest: Potential Recommendations

Case of Jason: Assessment Status Update

In addition to the various interventions that you have recommended for Jason, he has been through a medicine change and on beta interferon is now actually able to function between 32 to 40 hours during the work week. His gait has improved to some degree. He is taking trazadone and has less difficulty sleeping. His father is retiring, however, and he is within a few months of being "cut off" from his $1,000 a month stipend through his father's real estate group for consultative work. He truly needs to make greater progress relative to competitive work activity.

One of the services that you requested as part of the vocational assessment process was a neuropsychological evaluation. Jason's neuropsychological evaluation is presented in Figure III-2. It is of interest that for an individual who has completed law school, he has a Full Scale IQ score of 91, which is on the cusp of the lower third of the population. Among the WAIS-R subtests, he is particularly compromised on Digit-Symbol (subtest score of 5), which suggests difficulties with cognitive efficiency (<10th percentile) also supported on the Symbol Digit Test. A review of his percentile scores on the Wechsler Memory Scale-Revised (WMS-R) suggests fluctuating performances for both verbal and visual reproductive memory. His performances are between the 16th and the 82th percentile, but decidedly poor for an individual who is a law school graduate. His error score on the Booklet Category Test (74) is substantially worse than normal limits (> 50 errors), suggesting difficulties with abstraction and executive functioning. His score on the Tactual Performance Test was not available because the test was discontinued as he exceeded the time limits. This suggests difficulties with marked sensory perceptual problem solving (note, however, that the testee is blindfolded and does not benefit from vision). His performance on other tests such as Trails and D-2 also indicate significantly compromised cognitively flexibility and concerns with divided attention.

WAIS-R

VIQ	95
PIQ	88
FSIQ	91
Info	10
DS	10
Vocab	10
Anth	8
Comp	10
Sim	10
PC	8
PA	10
BD	9
QA	9
DSym	5

Stroop

Words	115" (6)
Colors	320" (3)

WRAT-R	SS	%	GE
Read	110	75	12+
Spell	105	63	12+
Anth	84	14	8B

WCST Per Resp = 38

Correct	78
Errors	50
PersErrr	33
Categories	5

WMS Form R

	Raw	%tile
DS Forward	10	82
DS Backward	6	47
Log Mem I	25	47
Log Mem II	19	36
Vis Repro I	35	65
Vis Repro II	24	16
Max# Forward =		7
Max # Backward =		4
Verbal Mem Index:		95

D-2 Test

Total	233
Errors	1
%Errors	.43
Accuracy	232
Fluctuation	10
Distribution	0-1-0

Symbol-Digit

Written	29	/	31
Oral	33	/	33

Halstead-Reitan Test Battery

Booklet

Category: I II   Total: 74

1 0   2 1   3 34   4 24
5 5   6 3   7 7

TPT: I II   III

Dom	10.3(10)
NDom	dc'ed
Both	Not admin
Seashore Rhythm	27 (Rank=31)
Speech Sounds	2
Tapping:	
NonDom	39.8
Dom	44.8

Impairment Index

Trails A	43"	(0)
Trails B	119"	(0)
Total	262"	(…)

FIGURE III-2   Jason's Neuropsychological Profile

A review of the testing indicates that Jason's strength is in his verbal skills. His arithmetic performances on the WAIS-R and the Wide Range Achievement Test-Revised are also poor for a college graduate. His rote attention and concentration reviewed on the Wechsler Memory Scale-Revised, the Seashore Rhythm, and Speech

Sounds Perception Test appear within a reasonable range. In general, he is going to require a position that is well structured, does not involve a high degree of cognitive efficiency and strong problem solving, and capitalizes on his past life experience and verbal skills. Jason is also a physically attractive male who dresses and presents well, which is a plus in the work setting.

Input from the vocational evaluation indicates recommendations related to semiskilled customer service work that is highly structured, has a modulated pace, and capitalizes on his language capabilities (e.g., describing available mortgage programs, responding to book orders, providing insurance quotes describing the benefits of available mutual funds within a company, etc.).

Recommending a Placement Approach for Jason

Now consider the vocational direction information from the neuropsychological report and Jason's medical stability (remission of significant MS exacerbations). Jason can sit with occasional standing over a full workday of six to eight hours and with some frequency is restricted to under-medium lifting—less than 30 pounds. Please take time to review and consider the following questions:

Questions and Answers Regarding Jason's Placement Plan (Facilitator initially uses only questions)

- Can we recommend one or more of the placement approaches in the Figure III-1 diagram at this time?

  Although it may be possible to start Jason immediately on a customer service job with a job coach or paid coworker as support, this may not be wise because of the dramatic fluctuations in his neuropsychological profile—the unevenness of his cognitive abilities presents questions as to capability.
- If immediate placement is not optimal, what type of service might be considered at this time?

Community-based assessment related to Jason's areas of interest utilizing the 215-hour Department of Labor waiver is probably in his best interests. Initially, he still wanted to utilize his law degree. Consequently, a community-based assessment was set up within the legal department of a Seattle medical research facility. Jason was not able to grasp the nature of assignments or their nuances and complexities despite significant mentoring and time allowance. Legal work in which he had full-service responsibility is unlikely.

- If or when ready to recommend a placement approach, with the position of a structured customer service job as the job goal, what type of placement avenue(s) might be used?

When the rehabilitation agency was ready to place Jason, it appeared that he most likely would benefit from a natural support, or a paid coworker as trainer.

- Might more than one placement approach be used?

The answer to this question is yes. It was in his best interests to be both selectively placed or brokered by the rehabilitation agency and then the paid coworker established as a mentor and on-the-job monitor. Either approach alone probably is insufficient for job stabilization.

- If assistive technology were to be employed, what type of procedural recommendations, work site physical modifications, or assistive equipment might be useful?

Assistive technology can be helpful in Jason's case. Particularly due to the memory problems, he might benefit from checklists, taping supervisor instructions, and using a self-evaluation protocol to check completed work product. Due to heat, he would also benefit from air conditioning in his place of employment.

Discussion Notes

Actual Placement Outcome

In working toward competitive placement with Jason, it was considered of mutual importance by both Jason (as the client) and his counselor that he try out structured legal work or paralegal work in the community while he tried again to pass the bar. He consequently did a three-month tryout within the legal department of a major research institute in the Seattle area. He simply was not able to initiate or organize legal activities with any consistency despite substantial mentoring. A second paralegal position within a law firm was similarly unsuccessful. Legal work activity appeared simply too complex and "rapid-fire" for Jason to adapt. He was also uncomfortable with the competitive work environment for the legal work. Unfortunately, despite extended time, a separate testing room, and other accommodations, Jason also was continually unable to pass the Washington state bar, which he had continued to pursue. The door was finally closed on legal pursuits and he was open to customer service activity.

At this juncture Jason, in some emotional "denial," decided to leave our vocational services project and tried three different placements on his own—claims work within a large managed care company, a "rapid-fire" customer service book order desk position, and again some work in a company legal department. In coming back to the project, he did indicate that job site support would be important. He was brokered by a placement specialist to an area equipment company and hired in customer service. This was done with a supervisor as a paid coworker. The supervisor worked with him on lunch hours and after hours, mentoring him in relation to procedures and helping him to develop a self-evaluation checklist. Accommodation at the work site was important during the warm summer months because he would fatigue, and an air-conditioning unit was purchased by the State Division of Vocational Rehabilitation. Jason was able to sustain the job for 18 months, when he was laid off as a result of a company change of ownership. He came back to the rehabilitation agency to seek other work, and he was subsequently referred to a call center position—again computer-based customer service work but with a modulated work flow. He was able to maintain this position with the help of a paid coworker mentoring him over time.

The placement model therefore was a combination of sequential direct or selectively brokered placement with paid coworker support. Although successful at this juncture, Jason may again need the assistance of a rehabilitation agency in the future. Fortunately, he has worked through some of the emotional denial relative to his capabilities and is open and aware of the need for support for coping strategies to shore up his cognitive deficits. Partially due to family of origin issues and expectations, he may vacillate in relation to disability denial—this may be an ongoing counseling issue.

References

Crewe, N and Athelston, G. (1984). Personal Capacities Questionnaire. Menomonee, WI: University of Wisconsin–Stout Materials Development Center.

Curl, R.M., Fraser, R.T., Cook, R.G., and Clemmons, D.C. (1996). Traumatic brain injury rehabilitation: Preliminary findings for the co-worker as trainer project. *J Head Trauma Rehabil* 11:75–85.

Curl, R.M., McConaughy, E.K., Pawley, J.M., and Salzberg, C.L. (1987a). Put that person to work! A coworker training manual for the coworker transition model. Logan, Utah: Utah State University Press.

Curl, R.M. and Hall, S.M. (1990). Put that person to work! A manual for implementors using the coworker transition model. Logan, Utah: Utah State University Press.

Curl, R.M., Mconaughy, E.K., Pawley, J.M., and Salzberg, C.L. (1987b) Put that person to work! A coworker training video for the coworker transition model [film]. Logan, Utah: Utah State University Press.

Curl, R.M., McConaughy, E.K., Pawley, J.M., and Salzberg, C.L. (1987c). Trainer and worker implemented tools [film]. Logan, Utah: Utah State University Press.

Fraser, R.T., Cook, R., Clemmons, D.C., and Curl, R.H. (1997). Work access in traumatic brain injury rehabilitation. *Phys Med Rehabil Clin North Am* 8:371–387.

Goldberg, R. (1992). Toward a model of vocational development of people with disabilities. *Rehabil Couns Bull* 35:161–173.

Gulick, E.E. (1987). Parsimony and model confirmation of the ADL Self-Care Scale for Multiple Sclerosis Persons. *Nurs Res* 40:107–112.

Herth, K (1992). Abbreviated instrument to measure hope. *J Adv Nurs* 17:1251–1259.

Kurtzke, J.F. (1983). Rating neurological impairment in multiple sclerosis: An expanded disability status scale (EDSS). *Neurology* 33:144–1452.

LaRocca, N. (1995). *Employment and multiple sclerosis.* New York: National Multiple Sclerosis Society.

Mendelsohn, S.B. Tax benefits and work incentives. In R.D. Rumrill, Jr. (ed.). *Employment issues and multiple sclerosis.* New York: Demos.

Minden, S.L. and Schiffler, R.B. (1990). Affective disorders in multiple sclerosis: Review and recommendations for clinical research. *Arch Neurol* 47:98–104.

National Multiple Sclerosis Society. (1997). Project Alliance final report. Funded by the Rehabilitation Services Administration, U.S. Department of Education, Washington, D.C., grant PR #H235H20001.

Roessler, R.T. (1996). The role of assessment in enhancing the vocational success of people with MS. *Work* 6:191–201.

Roessler, R. and Gottcent, J. (1994). The Work Experience Survey: A reasonable accommodation/career development strategy. *J Appl Rehabil Couns* 25:16–21.

Rubin, S. and Roessler, R. (1995). *Foundations of the vocational rehabilitation process.* Austin, TX: Pro-Ed.

Rumrill, P., Fraser, R., and Anderson, J. (2000). New directions in home-based employment for people with disabilities. *Journal of Vocational Rehabilitation*, 14:3–4.

Rumrill, P.D. (1996). Employment and multiple sclerosis: Policy, programming and research recommendations. *Work* 6:205–209.

Storey, K. and Certo, N.J. (1996). National supports for increasing integration in the workplace for people with disabilities: A review of the literature and guidelines for implementation. *Rehabil Couns Bull* 40:62–76.

Verdier-Taillefer, M.H. (1995). Occupational environment as risk factor for unemployment in MS. *Acta Neurol Scand* 92:59–62.

Wehman, P., Bricout, J., and Targett, P. (2000). Supported employment for persons with traumatic brain injury: A guide for implementation. In R.T. Fraser and D.C. Clemmons (eds.). *Traumatic brain injury rehabilitation: Practical vocational, neuropsychological, and psychotherapy interventions.* Boca Raton: CRC Press.

Psychosocial Issues and Interventions

Francie Bennett, M.S.W.

Most emotional responses to multiple sclerosis (MS) are normal reactions to a long-term and unpredictable illness. MS can impact a few to possibly all aspects of personal and interpersonal functioning (see Table IV-1). Emotional reactions can include clinical and subclinical levels of anxiety and reactive depression. Self-esteem may deteriorate. Grief reactions such as anger, denial, and sadness are likely to occur (Burnfield and Burnfield, 1982). The individual's and family's journey needs to include not only acceptance, however, but also often a series of emotional, behavioral, spiritual, intellectual, and social transformations—which accommodate the new subtle or dramatically changing realities of ongoing life with MS (Kalb, 1998; Strong, 1989). "Family" refers to whoever is identified as primary-level intimates or dependents, be they legal relatives or purely chosen.

Strong emotional responses may, in turn, alter the self-care and interpersonal behavior of the individual and the family coping with MS. Each exacerbation presents a degree of risk for a crisis reaction, depending, of course, on the individual, family, or other support systems (LeMaistre, 1985; Simons, 1984). Crisis reactions are prolonged or unsuccessfully resolved when preexisting coping mechanisms are overwhelmed, inadequate, or dormant. The knowledge that symptoms can reappear or that dramatic new symptoms and lifestyle alter-

TABLE IV-1   Potential Problems
■ Diminished energy, focus, and accomplishment
■ Displaced feelings (e.g., anger, fear)
■ Inappropriate behavior distracts/disturbs others
■ Communication and relationships deteriorate
■ Social factors deteriorate desirable level of functioning
■ Social withdrawal, alienation, rejection/abandonment
Also
■ Potential parenting problems may impact on other functioning

ations can occur increases the likelihood of anxiety and a wild ride of grief reaction each time the person and family encounter disease-related changes.

Family members are seldom in tandem in their grief reaction or knowledge of the disease. Preexisting personal or interpersonal problems are more likely to resurface or to be magnified during crisis periods. There is often an enhanced need for a social systems approach to effectively address the dynamic multilayered challenges.

Grief Reactions

There are a number of different grief reactions that can occur or reoccur with new exacerbations. Grieving may include one, a few, or all of the following manifestations (see Table IV-2):

- Shock—The person is temporarily overwhelmed and unable to connect feelings and information. The person might report, "It hasn't really sunk in yet," "I feel emotionally stunned," "in suspended animation," "numb," etc. This reaction is more common with the initial diagnosis and symptoms or with dramatically different and life-altering symptoms that may occur later in the disease's course.
- Denial—This defense can initially allow the person or family to postpone fully confronting what may be perceived to be

TABLE IV-2   Grief and Loss Roller Coaster Menu*
■ Shock
■ Denial
■ Flooding
■ Fear
■ Withdrawal
■ Sadness
■ Bargaining
■ Anger
■ Acceptance
■ Transformation

Combinations of the above can occur—Commonly activated with new MS exacerbations.

overwhelmingly frightening, radically alien, or shameful. Fatigue, for example, may be repeatedly minimized until the person feels like she or he has "hit a brick wall." Balance may deteriorate to the point where the person is bumping into furniture or falling down and yet even the informed person (or family) may cling to the explanation that this is due to "just clumsiness" or "not paying attention." Cognitive problems may be minimized or denied completely.

This becomes difficult, of course, when the denial persists, jeopardizing quality of life and safety or negatively affecting others. Denial or minimizing a problem can protract the development of adaptive behavior (e.g., using a cane or declining overly strenuous social activities). Altering behavior often requires problematic internal and social adjustments (e.g., for self-concept and social "normality"). Negative social and economic consequences make emergence from denial even less palatable.

It is important to remember that a person with MS, the person's family members, coworkers, and others may have very different information and come to grips with this disease at varying speeds. Others, including professionals, who are further down the path of disability acceptance may become frustrated and judgmental with a person who is still in denial or who appears to deny reality. Denial is not to be confused with anosagnosia or euphoria, neurologically induced problems that functionally resemble denial.

■ Fear—In a dominant culture obsessed with the concept of personal "independence," loss of the ability to be "independent" and "in control" may feel even more catastrophic. Also threatened are self-concept; the securing of pleasure; social regard; affection; the ability to tangibly care for dependents; one's livelihood, etc.

Because MS symptoms have the potential to be wide-ranging and dire, it is understandable that one can catastrophize or simply (and appropriately) try to anticipate, in efforts to protect oneself and loved ones (Brooks and Matson, 1987). A person may attempt to reinstate a sense of control by insatiably seeking information on MS, treatments, options, or even by becoming hypercontrolling in unrelated aspects of their life.

Depending on ethnic background, gender, socialization, and one's belief/behavior matrix, a person may express fear as anger or through other varying cultural or idiosyncratic responses. People with a history of abuse or neglect may experience exceptional fear of loss of control, dependency, and/or pain. Fear is powerful as both ally and tormentor.

■ Sadness—It is very normal to feel sad about real or potential (MS) losses for oneself and/or loved ones, about a reduced sense of security, or lost dreams, curtailed pleasures, or options and expectations. Some may encounter a sense of their mortality for the first time, ushering in important adjustments. For some individuals, the sorrow combined with pessimism and an overall excessive stress load can grow into a significant level of depression.

■ Bargaining—Some people will make an attempt to buy time or reasonable health by "being good" or making a sacrifice (e.g., through one's religion or spiritual "powers," or overcompliance with health care providers' recommendations or experimental treatments). A child may attempt to bargain for the parent's health by "being good," particularly younger children who may believe that they caused the disease or exacerbation(s).

- Anger—This is sometimes directed at the disease or sometimes displaced (e.g., toward family members, coworkers, doctors, "God," the person with MS, etc.). Within the family, anger may be directed at another member's grief behaviors or at the wellness of other family members and other support system members.

  Fear heightens anger. Anger may result when a person believes he or she is being treated in a cavalier manner while particularly vulnerable and at the other's mercy. Many people are quite uncomfortable receiving or witnessing anger and may react with anger or more subtle rejecting behavior when the "sender" is in the greatest need of support.

  Anger at health care providers, family members, etc. may simply be situation-specific and proportional (e.g., at a doctor for not allowing time for questions, at a spouse for not following up on a commitment). Grief-related anger should also not be confused with neurologically induced impulse control problems or preexisting psychological propensities for anger outbursts, etc.

- Withdrawal—Grieving (and otherwise adapting) may consume some time and energy previously focused elsewhere, resulting in withdrawal. The person or family may not be able to identify, communicate, or navigate this withdrawal behavior without assistance.

  Informal and formal support systems may pull away or be pushed away. They may react in various ways (e.g., condescension, lack of empathy, overt control) that emotionally if not physically isolate the "patient" or family. This may trigger anger. While some withdrawal may serve adjustment needs, and people's need for alone time varies, excessive withdrawal can ferment as well as represent depression.

- Guilt—A person with MS may feel guilt about "burdening" or "depriving" others due to the caregiving or support he or she needs; new role changes; diminished energy; lost income and lifestyle options, etc. Partners, coworkers, friends, and children may feel guilt about their own contrasting health and abilities, about leaving the person with MS out of activities, or about their own grief or resentments of the impact on their lives.

Partners, children, or other family can live with tremendous and secret guilt (and enormous stress) for years because they do not think that they "have the right" or that "it wouldn't be fair" to acknowledge their own needs. They may feel that they cannot acknowledge their own grief and needs because they do not "have the disease," fear personal censure, or fear that "it would hurt" others "to know how I feel." Some preexisting self-esteem problems or spiritual/belief systems heighten the risk of a guilt reaction (e.g., a "punishing God" or a more New Age belief that "I've invited this disease into my life and look at its impact on my family!").

- Acceptance—The individual and/or family members may not ever "embrace" the disease, but they may come to squarely acknowledge its symptoms, a need for coping "tools," or the disease in general. This paves the way for healthier adaptation. A person may be ready to accept and deal directly with a particular symptom, but not ready to fully accept all present and potential symptoms or the subsequent challenges in their life.

People can often only deal with so much at one time. A person coping fairly well with fatigue and using a cane, for example, may become overwhelmed and reactive to entering a room full of people with more severe MS or when reading about extreme symptoms. The steps and pacing to acceptance are very individual. Others, such as service providers, will need to practice respectful patience while supporting progress. Anosagnosia (neurologically based lack of awareness) can interfere with the recognition necessary to acceptance.

- Personal Reformulation (beyond grief)—This process often involves many elements, including absorbing and integrating information; time and experience; reframing of oneself and one's context; awareness of options and behaviors; identifying and utilizing adequate internal and external supports; flexibility; creativity; hope; assertiveness; pursuit of interests and pleasures; and positive thinking. A compassionate sense of humor is also tremendously helpful.

Many people will need to add to their preexisting life skills in order to truly thrive and not just survive with MS. The individual and family will do this in steps over time. Successful adaptation in one area of life, such as improved communication or creative problem solving in the family, will likely assist in other areas such as vocational adaptation. Successful experiments in living with new symptom realities breed the skill, confidence, and hope necessary to approach change elsewhere.

Many people with MS and their families have reported to this author that MS can serve a "teaching" function in their lives after some period of initial adjustment. They may learn, for example, to be more flexible, assertive, and creative in their problem solving; have a better sense of humor; clarify priorities; choose their "battles" more carefully; and to live with heightened appreciation of gifts of the moment. Neurologic compromise of cognitive and emotional functions can delay or alter the reformulation process (e.g., emotional/situational incongruency or the inability to remember insights or adaptive skills).

It is important to remember that not all problems are due to the long tentacles of MS (see Table IV-3). Pre-MS challenges with family,

---

TABLE IV-3   Other Problems

- Euphoria
- Emotional lability
- Schizophrenia
- Bipolar disorder
- Preexisting psychological and/or interpersonal dysfunction (e.g., PTSD, family crisis, bipolar disorder)
- Substance or physical abuse
- Somatic complaints

employer, or others can be prominent. People with preexisting problems such as rigidity, low self-esteem, or poor emotional integration will have a more difficult time transitioning. Alcohol and other addictions, abuse, or major mental health disorders will need to be well addressed before real progress can be made. Life goes on, and other problems are sure to present. Teenage mood swings, gardening backaches, mid-life crises, or other illnesses are possible and deserve differentiated care.

Emotional Triggers

In sufficient load, the items listed in Tables IV-4a and IV-4b can trigger and augment depression and anxiety for the person with MS.

Ritvo and coworkers (1992) note that MS patients scored worse than a normal population on the MHI (Mental Health Inventory) and that the best predictive model for mental health in MS includes the FIS (fatigue impact scores), perceived social support (revised UCLA Loneliness Scale), and duration of symptoms (collectively accounting for 68 percent of variance in the MHI scores). It is notable that the FIS alone accounted for 38 percent of the variance in MHI scores. Provinciali and coworkers (1999) note depression's score increasing as independent of any physical or cognitive disability, but view depression as primarily related to fatigue.

MS fatigue can be profound and undermine multiple aspects of lifestyle. It is one of the "invisible" symptoms that is often misunderstood and inappropriately judged by others. An increase in MS fatigue can trigger some emotional reactions that make everything harder. For example, let's consider an individual who has afternoon fatigue, which is very common for people with MS. If he or she is working or spending time with family in the afternoon and "hits the wall" and needs to rest, the person may feel guilty and less worthy or may feel more depressed and hopeless. "Will I ever get over this fatigue?" "Will I ever be able to live my life again?" The depression that the person may have, either clinically or subclinically, can of course also reduce general activity and quality of life levels. One can have both an emotional fatigue

---

TABLE IV-4A   Depression Triggers

- Grief and loss
- Sense of powerlessness
- Sense of hopelessness
- Insufficient or inactive coping mechanisms
- Insufficient or underutilized supports
- Social triggers (e.g., abuse, abandonment, discrimination)
- Physically induced (brain chemistry or lesions)
- Medication side effects or medication management problems
- Idiosyncratic reactions to medications

TABLE IV-4B   Anxiety Contributors

- "Unpredictability" of future
- Sense of impending catastrophes
- Sense of powerlessness
- Inability to meet basic needs for self and dependents
- Insufficient or inactive coping mechanisms
- Insufficient or underutilized supports
- Social triggers (e.g., abuse, threat of abandonment, "isms")
- Physically induced (e.g., brain chemistry)
- Medication side effects or medication management problems
- Idiosyncratic reactions to medications
- Loss of lifestyle activities that pleasure, stimulate, and provide meaning
- Neurologic changes to cognition, mood, and behavior
- Anticipation of impending catastrophe
- Fatigue or pain

---

and a physically based fatigue. Fatigue, depression, and isolation can heighten pain perception and decrease concentration and memory.

People with MS often say that they could better manage the problems and symptoms that MS brings if they had more energy. Therefore, assessing the cause of the fatigue is important. Antidepressants can decrease some fatigue. There are also some other medications (e.g., amantadine) that help some (but not all) people with the fatigue generated by the MS itself. A medical consultation for differentiating assessment and treatment is highly recommended. An occupational therapist can be very helpful in tailoring energy conservation strategies with the individual. A psychotherapist may be able to assist the person to grieve, prioritize, and balance needs with available energy.

Depression may tend to magnify concerns and the subjective perception of symptoms in MS. It is sometimes confusing to sort out depression from the actual symptoms of MS because some of them are identical or very similar. Chronic fatigue with problems in concentration, memory, and task completion can give the appearance of depression when it's not present. Cognitive problems may also be misattributed to the MS, but often will actually clear as depression or anxiety dissipate. Magnified attention to and the experience of pain and other symptoms may result from depression, but also from decreased external stimuli as people withdraw in order to conserve their own energy. The fatigue that is common in MS can frequently be differentiated from the fatigue in depression because MS-specific fatigue is stimulated by heat and physical exertion, generally worsening in the afternoon. Fatigue fostered by depression may be worse earlier in the day or remain fairly constant.

Family and Significant Others

Poor information and lack of support often leads unnecessarily to family stress (see Table IV-5). For example, it's often hard for family members to understand the fatigue levels experienced by a person with a disability. They may not have the information necessary to really acknowledge and support the person when they are fatigued. They may think or say the person "looks just fine," "maybe they're just lazy," "maybe they're depressed," and so forth. This avoidable misperception can breed censure, resentment, and alienation at a time when clarity and supportive problem solving are most needed.

There can be significant role changes. A child, partner, or aging parent often becomes a long-term caregiver in varying degrees. In the case of children, this may ultimately influence their personality devel-

TABLE IV-5 Family Responses (also relevant for close friend or coworkers)

- Grief and loss reactions
- Poor information leads to avoidable family stress
- Potential role changes
- Caregiver burnout potential
- Potential loss of childhood for the young caregiver/ impairing personality development
- Kids may act out
- Often undersupported spouse/significant other
- "Secrets" develop: Guilt, resentment, and living separate lives
- Preexisting problems magnified

opment, risking their becoming "overly helpful" personalities. They may miss some of the childhood experiences that they need while taking care of parents and assuming other responsibilities. Certainly children can take care of other family members and home care to some degree, but there is a point at which it may become too much. Young people can emotionally respond to both the MS and their lack of information and sophistication about it by feeling guilty or angry, by acting out at school or home, or by having fears, depression, or anxiety of their own. Grief, sometimes expressed in other terms, is not uncommon with children. A scared, angry child acting this out at school can also be a powerful distraction to the parent struggling to accommodate significant MS changes while at work. Children's negative reactions to MS can be reduced by assuring them it is not their fault, minimizing effects on their lifestyle, and generally maintaining healthy communication and parenting patterns within the family.

A worn-out, secretly resentful, or depressed spouse or significant other with caregiving responsibilities may not be able to provide the support that the person with MS needs in order to perform optimally at work or in other arenas. Certainly spouses and significant others have their own issues with MS (and other aspects of their life!). They may not feel free to talk with the person who has MS, or in fact anyone, "because," after all, they "don't have MS." This can lead to hidden feelings of "burn-out," anger and resentment, and tremendous guilt. Caregivers can suffer crushing emotional problems such as depression and fatigue because of the long-term caregiving proposition and losses in meeting their own needs adequately.

The couple may have substantial role changes during exacerbations or as the disease progresses. Role changes need to be addressed. If one partner becomes too much of "the caregiver" and the other person "the patient," the health of the marriage is at risk. MS, itself, can affect sexual functioning in numerous ways (e.g., pain, fatigue, reduced erection, sensation, etc.). Reactive emotions can certainly also affect how people respond sexually. Those consuming all their energy at work or as caregiver at home may not be able to rise above exhaustion or resentment in order to enjoy quality time with spouse. Intimacy and desire in general can deteriorate as care giving, fatigue, and emotional reactions to the changes and challenges diminish desire and opportunity. Creative solutions to MS-induced impotence, painful intercourse, or incontinence might otherwise be explored.

A troubled primary relationship is also likely to impact work. From a vocational rehabilitation standpoint, a family systems approach to assessment and intervention can be critical for improving vocational goal attainment.

Community Reactions

Discrimination toward anyone "different" in our society is easily and observably targeted toward people with disabilities. Respectful and caring inclusion in the everyday life of the community for people with disabilities is fairly new and incomplete. Fortunately, many negative reactions can be ameliorated through informal and formal education and advocacy. Legal approaches are important, but the bulk of social and economic progress is still likely to come about through other and less formal means.

Sometimes whole formal and informal support systems pull apart (see Table IV-6). Friends and coworkers do sometimes pull away or are pushed away by the person with MS. It is not uncommon for people to feel some discomfort and to exhibit avoidance, conde-

TABLE IV-6 Community Reactions

- Often mis- or underinformed about disease
- Society teaches stereotypes and discriminates
- Little counterbalancing experience
- Often quite difficult to understand invisible symptoms ("You look so good" syndrome)
- Fear
- Discomfort, avoidance, or overcompensation
- Often educable and open to positive influence

scension, overprotection, or other overcompensatory behavior. The shadow of the "disability closet" is still close by, and people remain "green" at intellectually and behaviorally appropriate responses to those with disabilities. If the foundation of a job or peer group interaction were defined rather singularly—for example, by a lot of physical activity and prowess—and the person with MS needs to modify these activities, she can lose some social contacts, status, support, and vocational options. In this example, friends may also need time to examine and broaden their sense of a person's worth and sources of enjoyment. Dialogue between the person with MS and peer group discussing members' beliefs, feelings, specific MS symptoms, and adaptive options can often improve negative reactive relationships over time. The person with MS will often need to initiate and try to set the tone for this dialogue.

An employer may be concerned about meeting production deadlines and retaining a valued employee. Employers may also not understand how they can work within the Americans with Disabilities Act (ADA) guidelines without significant cost or operational upheaval in their businesses. Information for employers or community members about this disease and tailored response models can be crucial. Ancillary vocational issues are explored further in a later section entitled "Psychosocial Issues in Vocational Success." Categories of work-related accommodation are reviewed in Section III of this book.

Communities (as well as people with MS and their family) can have a difficult time with fatigue; bladder and bowel problems;

changes in cognitive function; and general "personality" characteristic changes. Pronounced emotional or behavioral changes, either induced by the MS itself or as emotional reactions to the MS, can profoundly affect relationships.

Fatigue for the person with MS can shorten or abruptly end social discourse, work, and other desirable activities within the community. This can be not only frustrating for all involved but often misunderstood because of ignorance and the belief that the person with MS often "looks just fine."

Symptoms such as bladder or bowel control can have profound impact on a person's comfort and to some degree the ability to function in the community—in part, because of the psychosocial, as well as practical, response to these problems. Pads or catheters are often only adapted to after psychological anguish and resistance due to personal and societal standards, competing reinforcers, and discrimination perceptions have been resolved.

Personality propensities are often poorly understood in general. More dramatic alterations in cognition or emotionaland behavioral patterns in a friend, customer, or employee can be perceived and treated as an unpredictable threat. Community members may be slower to adjust to the complexities of behavioral changes than to other more tangible elements of MS.

Tailored information about the disease and treatment or coping options can help to "normalize" responses, empower all concerned, and make neurologic problems seem more manageable (see Table IV-7). It is important to note that people tend to become less overwhelmed when information is presented regarding symptoms they personally experience.

Fortunately, community contacts, employers, and families are often very educable, but we do need to provide information. The individual who has MS may benefit from learning how to educate other people. Sometimes behavioral rehearsal of an MS educational presentation to employers and loved ones is useful. Handouts and materials about MS can also be helpful. Support and role modeling, through others with the disability or other allies, can bolster the courage and skills needed for community activism, advocacy, and education.

TABLE IV-7   Interpersonal Matrix
■ Synergistic effect of combined social responses
■ Poor information, attitude, or communication promotes misunderstanding and dysfunction that breeds downward cycle
■ Stereotypes breed anger and fear which also magnify other problems
■ Mutual respect and open creative discovery help build positive solutions
■ Problems and solutions in one area of life have a way of spilling over into the workplace
■ Not everything is due to MS!
■ MS can also be a teacher

Problem resolution in one area of life may have a way of spilling over into the workplace. As the person who has MS and his or her family learn more about this disability, they can become more comfortable, self-esteem can be reestablished or improved for the person with the disability, and coping mechanisms can be strengthened, reinforced, or returned to a more natural state. This, in turn, has a way of affecting the person's functioning and self-presentation within the community, including at the work site.

Family members may be in critical need of support and assistance, but are often underserved in the health care environment which focuses on "the MS patient." This seems symptomatic of our society's myopic difficulty in seeing the interconnectedness of the web of life. A societal paradigm shift is probably required for substantial change but families and social workers may seek family inclusion on a case by case basis in the meantime.

Interaction of Psychosocial Issues and Neuropsychological Status

The neuropsychological changes caused by MS can have a ripple effect in the patient's life and in the lives of others around him. Others often respond negatively to an individual who, for example, due to MS lability or euphoria, is frequently laughing or crying or whose life perspectives, daily functioning, and emotional responses are otherwise inappropriate. An employer may have trepidation about consequent impact on customers, other employees, and general performance. Friends and coworkers may feel awkward or alienated and become more reticent to interact or may react nonconstructively.

An individual with an MS-induced euphoria may appear to have odd, mismatched emotional reactions or not be able to appropriately connect with what is occurring in his or another's life. For example, one man recovering from this condition told the author that he had not grieved for an extended period when a favorite relative died. His apparent indifference was seen as heartlessness by his family. A health care provider, if aware of this condition, could have helped him and his family sort out and adapt to the problem.

A person who is having word accessing problems, slurred speech, and difficulty remembering important work and family data, or who is displaying emotional dyscontrol due to the MS, is likely to encounter adjustment issues not only within herself, but also within family and community contexts.

Neurologic changes can alter functional capacities and personality significantly or in rather subtle and minor ways. Some can be compensated for in concrete ways such as memory aids. Some losses require adaptation in a primarily social, intellectual, or an emotional fashion (such as education of others about neurologically based lability). The potential for complex and changing symptoms further complicates personal and interpersonal adjustment.

The individual who has MS symptoms such as slurred speech, diminished concentration, poor balance, or gait problems may feel very embarrassed about going out in public. She may fear that other people will view her as inebriated or otherwise socially less acceptable. Consequently, individuals may go out of the home less or socialize less. They may become more withdrawn, which in turn promotes depression and physical deterioration. Indeed a person's life has changed, but it's changed even more because of the very natural and understandable emotional reaction to these changes.

The recognition of cognitive function changes were historically often avoided and poorly understood even by many physicians. Estimates of the number of people affected cognitively as a result of MS vary, as discussed in Section II. Some of the changes that may need to be evaluated include attention, short-term memory, abstraction, speed of information processing, decision making, word naming, or the ability to multitask or set priorities.

Now family members who report "I'm seeing memory and decision making problems that he didn't have before," are much more likely to have that observation affirmed. This is very helpful because the family can then begin adapting rather than denying or polarizing. Understanding that the deficits are neurologic, not a reflection of character, can make them more psychologically and socially palatable. This can help pave the way for accommodations that may include role changes within the family or at the work site. An individual who was relied on at work or at home to do bookkeeping, make financial decisions, or set financial priorities may not be aware that these functional capacities have changed. Family, or others frequently around him may be a better source of information than the person with the cognitive disability. Sometimes family members need a safe or professionally facilitated environment to initiate discussions about delicate matters, such as loss of cognitive abilities. For example, a person with MS may buy impulsively, not remember the list of things that one would normally remember at the store, wind up buying a bunch of things to overcompensate, get overstimulated and emotionally distracted, frustrated and irritated, and have emotional outbursts that were not present before. One wonderfully creative and loving family I knew reduced the sense of shame involved in such incidents by softly joking that the MS "Bubba" had taken over at such times.

Persons who were, for example, weaker in skills such as financial management (but contributed in other significant ways within the family or at the work setting) may find themselves now taking on additional functions with some stress, confusion, or resentment.

A person may find some adaptations that enable him or her to continue at least parts of prior roles. She may decide, for example, "I'm going to do my more cognitively demanding tasks earlier in the day when I feel more focused." Adaptive retention of roles can enhance a person's sense of hope, a sense of increasing one's personal power and control, which is so at risk with long-term chronic illness.

The individual who has difficulty in cognitive functioning (e.g., concentration and task completion when they are overly stimulated by the environment) may need to work in a more isolated situation. As a result he may avoid social interaction at work which would, however, otherwise provide some pleasure, provide stimulus for improved self-esteem, and social support. Compensatory strategies may be required (e.g., making lunch more of a social event with colleagues).

People who have MS and their close family members often report that increasing emotional distress tends to activate or enhance MS symptoms, but studies remain inconclusive. Decreased environmental distractions, diminished emotional and intellectual stimulation, and curtailed pleasurable activities can amplify one's perception of pain, much as looking down a funnel will enhance one's perception of a reduced field of vision. Vegetative behavior common to depression or illness also impacts the body in ways that increase pain and therefore call attention to the body. Chronic pain increases the risk of depression and suicidal ideation. People with depression often report higher levels of pain for specific problems than people without depression. Distress does create changes in the body, which may make it indeed more difficult for the body to cope with illness. One's socialization patterns (e.g., gender, ethnicity, religion) can also foster variety in the experience, interpretation, and reporting of symptoms and the identification of stressors. Conclusions about synergistic factors of health and emotions seem as varied as facets of a prism in our society at this time.

Profound impulsive emotional outbursts or behavioral dyscontrol are sometimes symptomatic of a less common neurologic alteration. Hypersexuality, impulsive buying or traveling, and other such manic mood symptoms should be assessed for possible bipolar disorder or other brain dysfunction. A neuropsychiatrist can be key in this type of differential diagnosis.

Lack of relevant knowledge can leave a patient or others assuming that the person has become psychotic or hysterical. Neurologic damage can create some unusual symptoms such as the sensation of bugs crawling on skin. Historically, patients with MS were too often misdiagnosed with psychiatric disorders. Women with transitory or nonobservable symptoms were all too frequently not believed regarding their physical concerns (being viewed as hysterical, attention-seeking, depressed, etc.) and provided with psychiatric services only. This is rapidly declining as the use of magnetic resonance imaging (MRI) and its interpretation becomes more sophisticated and available. It is now firmly established that there is clearly no "MS personality." Thankfully, that debate has largely disappeared. Similarities and differences between neurologically versus psychosocially related fatigue and cognitive compromise were already addressed in the subsection on emotional triggers. Professionals and family alike need to stay humbly aware of their own preferences and biases toward neurologic versus psychosocial explanations.

Information about the causes of role changes and options for problem resolution can be very empowering to everybody involved. This input can give hope, helping the family adjust and adapt to changes that may be very stressful. Professionals providing intervention have a very important role to play in minimizing shame and other stresses while maximizing options and supporting proactive responses.

Murray (1995) observes that "Neurologists may find it difficult at times to recognize neuropsychological impairments when they see a patient in their office because changes present at that time can be subtle and the person may appear quite normal." Family members often can be very helpful in observing and reporting changes that the person who has the disability may not recognize or report.

Counseling Issues and Strategies

Without assistance in coming to terms with the MS and its changes, an individual may have a very difficult time maintaining positive self-esteem, socializing adequately, moving through grief, or breaking the spiral of depression and anxiety (Murray, 1995). The neurologic impact on cognitive functions and personality can further complicate emotional and behavioral responses (Murray, 1995). This in turn affects functioning at work or home, in the community, and with support systems in general.

Quality of life studies on people with MS indicate a number of factors that tend to affect mental health and quality of life: fatigue, loneliness and companionship, degree of chronic pain, duration of symptoms, other stressful life events, and cognitive deficits (Murray, 1995) (see Table IV-8). The neurologic disability may be less impairing to people with MS than the social isolation, inadequate communication and support, and the related psychosocial factors that they experience. Fatigue, grief, and other factors that can compromise social support and quality of life have been addressed earlier.

Because most people do not have pre-MS experience with disability, compensatory coping mechanisms need to be adapted and reinforced, or new ones developed. MS symptoms may "push" people beyond their preexisting coping levels. Heightened adjustment to chronic disease is very challenging, but often manageable (Murray, 1995). Those with the disability and their families will benefit from a strong network of support, counseling, and education. Psychotherapists may integrate all three elements in their work.

An individual often needs counseling assistance in order to strengthen or reactivate preexisting coping mechanisms and to build new ones as deficits are identified. Critical coping mechanisms can include: reaching out for and utilizing social support systems; self-nurturance and comforting; creative problem solving skills; a good sense of humor; and accessing of strong spiritual or philosophical beliefs that help to give hope and comfort. The potential for complex and changing symptoms further complicates personal and interpersonal adjustment. It is critical that one not only accept the loss and change, but also actually transform one's life to meet the realities of the disease and capitalize on remaining and new options.

Another coping mechanism is the ability to live in the present and to proactively deal with what's in front of one rather than anticipating catastrophes in the future or obsessively dwelling on the losses of the past. Finding ways to enjoy one's life within the real parameters of the disability is very important and ameliorates the impact of depression and anxiety. Cognitive-behavioral strategies such as

TABLE IV-8   Psychological/Social Pulls

↑ Creative solutions	↑ Social support
↑ Flexibility	↑ Positive outlook
↑ Pre-existing strengths	↑ Self-care
↑ Maintaining sense of humor	↑ Assertiveness
↑ Securing good information	↑ Communication
↑ Multidisciplinary health care	↑ Self-talk
↓ Grief experience	↓ Experience of discrimination
↓ Increased fatigue	↓ Feelings of loss of control
↓ Neurologic impairment of	↓ Financial instability
self-awareness, emotional	↓ Withdrawal/isolation
or behavioral control	
↓ Cognitive decline	

thought-stopping, attention focusing, setting manageable daily priorities, and brainstorming or experimentation with creative strategies can be very practical and useful gifts from therapy.

A positive attitude and hopefulness are very important in adapting to the changes wrought by this disease (Murray, 1995). People with positive spiritual or philosophical beliefs can find these to be a source of comfort and hope. People who have emotionally healthy supports may have hope because they know that they will have people there to help them adjust and cope both on a practical and on an emotional or spiritual level as they move through life. Counseling can reinforce and strengthen these supports through exploration, encouragement, and behavioral skill-building strategies.

Supportive counseling for grief (identifying, validating, and venting of feelings) may need to at least begin before exploration of additional coping mechanisms can proceed. Emotional flooding with sorrow or anger may leave no room for additional life changes or even activation of some familiar coping skills in the short run. Grief responses and other mental health concerns often vacillate with exacerbations and other social, psychological, and financial stressors as discussed earlier. Grief reactions need to be framed as generally normal. Identifying them as such offers important validation and comfort for people dealing with life change and loss. Assisting the person and her family to name and validate their grief responses paves the way to reclamation of coping mechanisms and supports healthy functioning. Depression, anxiety, and all of the grief reactions need to be looked for, assessed, and patiently and respectfully validated as the person and her family is helped to move through each occurrence (where internal and external support or skill are insufficient or more sophisticated health interventions are otherwise needed).

Carefully differentiated diagnoses should be made for symptoms that can be caused by more than one MS-related factor. For example, mania or depression symptoms can be caused by internal or external sources such as bipolar disorder or by medication problems such as steroid reactions.

Newer medications and progressive multidisciplinary approaches offer hope for improved physical and psychosocial functioning. Current medications provide many people with longer periods of relief or lighter symptoms when they do occur, as well as slower overall functional decline.

While there can be partial or total recovery, there is still the risk for some partial disability remaining during the remission phase of relapsing–remitting MS. But the hope is, of course, that it can be symptomatically inactive or plateau for months or years, or that a cure will be found. Remissions, even with a higher disability plateau (e.g., the lesions may still affect cognitive function), allow people to catch their emotional breath, stabilize, and adapt more easily than a progressive or pervasive decline pattern. The counselor has a critical role to play in supporting patients' medication trials and appropriate participation in allied health services such as speech, physical, and occupational therapies—as well as complementing health services such as massage.

Unfortunately, inpatient health care providers often see only the most difficult and advanced problems, potentially jading perspective and diminishing hope (Burnfield and Burnfield, 1982). The roles of hope and hope-giving and realistic encouragement by health care workers are very important. The person with MS and her family can benefit by being supported in their hope by other people, including a counselor with a positive perspective who is really equipped to deal with the sophisticated issues involved with MS.

As energy decreases and new priorities have to be set, a person's daily zone of activity may shrink. For example: a nurse with MS may have just enough energy to go to work and do her job, but she may not have the energy once she gets home to have quality time with her child, prepare dinner, or to take care of the home—let alone to socialize. Exploration of options that realistically accommodate priorities and psychosocial balance will be key to long term mental health.

Multiple sexual problems are triggered neurologically, emotionally, and interpersonally by MS (e.g., difficulties with arousal, libido, erection, or anorgasmia). Fatigue management and adaptive strategies for social or sexual problems can be important counselor and allied health care interventions. Combinations of medication, patient education, and skilled counseling can improve many except the most shallow or rigid of intimate sexual relationships.

While MS can certainly affect an individual's ability to work now and in the future, it still is important to note that a person with MS who continues to work will retain or is likely to have a stronger sense of self-esteem and a more positive, proactive approach to life. People with chronic progressive disease from the onset may watch employment options dwindle more quickly due to discrimination, escalated functional losses, and may lack the "luxury" of symptom plateaus and remissions in which to emotionally recharge and adjust. Counseling that helps to build or rebuild a positive view of a person and enhance options and skills (such as assertiveness) can aid the employment or successful retirement outlook.

Psychological support and information for the whole family is often critical and advisable. As symptoms increase, the demands on others often become greater. Caregivers are then at risk for problems with chronic sleep loss, insufficient rest, chronic fatigue, and certainly depression. If caregivers become ill or burn out, they may be less able to "pick up the pieces." This can affect the stress level of patients with MS and their ability to function in those areas that were being compensated for by the caregiver. MS must be considered a disability that affects the life of a caregiver, a spouse or significant other, the children, and anybody else intimately involved with the individual having the disability.

Sometimes separate counseling or groups, particularly for caregivers and spouses are needed. The caregiver, spouse, or children can vent some of their resentment and less pleasant feelings in a "safe" environment where they're not afraid of hurting or angering the person who has the disability. The individual and his or her family need to be assisted to activate appropriate supports for everyone impacted.

Counselors should have some experience with chronic illness of some kind. Lupus, for example, has some similar symptoms and problems. If counselors don't have any experience with MS or chronic illness then they need to be "quick learners." They need to be willing to educate themselves because there are some significant differences between the general healthy population and people who are coping with chronic illness. Nor is chronic illness support the same as grief support during death and dying processes.

Generally speaking, it is most advisable to connect people desiring psychotherapy with counselors who are cognitive-behavioral in their approach. Part of the challenge in counseling is to provide information or to support the individual and his family in accessing information—to generally assist individuals in increasing their awareness of self, others, and resources. Insight therapy, however, should be noted as often not appropriate for people with strong cognitive function difficulties. Memory retention deficits, abstraction problems, and the like, will undermine sustained progress, increase frustration, and diminish self-esteem and hopefulness. Some people with MS will function well with, and may prefer, more traditional models of therapy. Usually, however, a more active, interactive model that provides tailored education, coping strategies, behavioral rehearsal (including modifications of internal imagery and self-talk), along with grief and interpersonal support (and crisis intervention as needed) is more helpful. Memory aids may be critical to this work and clients should be allowed and encouraged to utilize recorders, notebooks, or homework handouts as needed during and between sessions. Asking clients, particularly those with known cognitive difficulties, to paraphrase or summarize key therapy points can be a helpful cross-check.

Community Referrals

It is important for counselors to know that a multidisciplinary approach is often very helpful, even critical. Physical therapy, occupational therapy, and speech therapy may also help an individual to increase actual physical functioning. This then strengthens their sense of self-worth, hope, personal power, independence, and so forth, thus providing significant psychological benefit. Specialized sexual advisement or counseling may be a referral need due to pain, spasming, sensation, bowel and bladder issues, or medication side effects. Counseling can support and encourage an individual to pursue an allied health therapy, set up an appointment, and follow through with prescribed treatment regimens in an area. The different disciplines can really work well together as a team and need to be encouraged to do so.

A counselor can also reinforce the work of the medical team by paying attention to and describing medication use and effects between doctor visits. This can be particularly helpful if a person with MS is unable to assess medication or treatment reaction, or if he tends to deny problems that are occurring (a patient "release of information" protocol needs to be carefully observed to maintain ethical and relationship integrity).

Peer support referrals, in the form of MS support groups appropriate to one's level of MS symptoms, can be psychologically helpful depending on the group and the individual involved. Some groups are comprised primarily of people who have greater levels of MS symptoms and may involve individuals who utilize wheelchairs and other assistive devices. A person who has milder symptoms may not function well and may be more prone to feel depressed in the midst of exposure to severe disability. Matching an individual to an appropriate peer support group or individual supportive peers is important.

Telephone networks need to be considered not only due to the nature of the disability, but lack of transportation and distance. Some community organizations may provide screening, sophisticated training, and supervision of peer support volunteers, but unfortunately this is not a norm.

For those individuals who have a computer and access to the Internet, there are also chat rooms for people with MS. There is a certain kind of empowerment that comes from connecting with other people who have similar symptoms (but who are hopefully not invested in having one necessarily select the same options or solutions they offer). This can be in addition to professional psychotherapy. Sometimes, an individual needs to search for a while to find the right match.

A caution, of course, related to peer support groups or for peer supporters (and for some professional counselors as well), is that "alternative" under-researched treatments may be encouraged by peers that have a negative impact on a person's financial resources, mood, or their actual health. There have been many controversial promotions of cures and interventions (which doesn't necessarily mean of course that they aren't of some help even as a placebo) including amalgam removal, snake venom treatments, certain psychic healing techniques, herbs, or bee stings.

An individual who selects a more alternative approach may want to have a discussion with a counselor about it. It is particularly critical to respect an individual's choices because MS often significantly threatens a person's sense of control and personal power. Assisting the person and her family to learn more about the disability, interventions, and cost/benefit analysis techniques can be very empowering. A counselor can explain the basics of how medical interventions are evaluated and help prepare the individual and her family for a discussion with a health care provider (e.g., a physician, nurse practitioner, naturopath, etc.) about potential benefits and risks. This may involve some assertion skills training. It may be useful for a counselor to educate or remind clients that MS symptoms may naturally diminish, stabilize, or go into remission, regardless of intervention. The patient with a plan and evaluative context within which to assess medications and interventions will simply be less anxious, vulnerable, depressed, and more confident.

Hope does play a part and there is a strong placebo effect in MS interventions. If an alternative treatment model doesn't bankrupt the person or if it doesn't harm the person physically, a person may wish to attempt it (because, for example, one "doesn't want to look back in 20 years and wish that they had tried something").

There is a certain sense of empowerment and hope in being involved with researching and fine tuning one's own interventions. Many people with MS, in the author's experience, educate themselves very well about the interventions and the costs and benefits of different interventions available in both the medical and alternative medicine arenas. Peer support networks and Internet sites are more likely to provide a wider range of information, opinion, and advice than that available through medical personnel.

Emotional support (and lots of advice!) can also be obtained through articles on the Internet and through quite a variety of books now on the market for coping with chronic illness or dealing specifically with MS. The National MS Society and some local MS organizations provide information and linkages to other resources. Some also offer MS specific counseling or other services, as well.

Recommended Reading

For professionals or people who are living with more advanced MS symptoms and are not frightened by frank in-depth discussions of topics such as bowel management (not everyone is comfortable with the scope): *Multiple Sclerosis:The Questions You Have–The Answers You Need*, 2nd ed., by Rosalind C. Kalb, Ph.D. (ed.), 2000, New York: Demos.

I would also recommend that counselors read the books *Mainstay* and *Beyond Rage* noted below. A useful book generally for mood management from a cognitive-behavioral standpoint is *Feeling Good—The New Mood Therapy*, by David D. Burns, M.D., 1980, New York: Penguin Group, Penguin Books, Inc.

For patients, families, or those interested in MS:

Beyond Rage, by JoAnn LeMaistre, Ph.D., 1985, Oak Park, Ill.: Alpine Guild.

Enabling Romance: A Guide to Love, Sex, and Relationships for the Disabled, K. Kroll, and E.L. Klein, 1992, New York: Harmony Books.

Fall Down Seven Times, Get Up Eight—Living Well With Multiple Sclerosis, J.D. Wolf, 1992, Rutland, VT: John K. Academic Books.

Living With Multiple Sclerosis: A Handbook For Families, R. Shuman, and J. Schwartz, 1994, New York: Collier Books.

Living With Multiple Sclerosis: A Wellness Approach, 2nd ed., by George Kraft, M.D., and Marci Catanzaro, R.N., Ph.D., 1999, New York: Demos.

Mainstay, by Maggie Strong, 1989, New York: Penguin Books.

Multiple Sclerosis: A Guide for Families, Rosalind C. Kalb, Ph.D., ed., New York: Demos, 1998.

Multiple Sclerosis: A Guide for the Newly Diagnosed, 2nd ed., N.J. Holland, T.J. Murray, and S.R. Reingold, 2001, New York: Demos Medical Publishing.

Multiple Sclerosis—A Self-Care Guide To Wellness, N. Holland and J. Halper, 1998, Washington, D.C.: Paralyzed Veterans of America.

My Mommy's Special, J. English, 1985, Chicago, Ill: Childrens Press.

Plaintalk. A Booklet About Multiple Sclerosis for Family Members, by Sarah L. Minden, M.D., and Debra Frankel, M.S., 1987, revised 1992, New York: National Multiple Sclerosis Society.

Self-Esteem: A Family Affair, by J.I. Clarke, 1978, New York: Harper Collins.

Sexuality and Intimacy in Multiple Sclerosis, F.W. Foley, in *Multuiple Sclerosis: A Guide for Families*, Rosalind C. Kalb, Ph.D., ed., New York: Demos, 1998.

Sexuality and Multiple Sclerosis, pamphlets from the National Multiple Sclerosis Society of the U.S. (New York) and the National Multiple Sclerosis Society of Canada (Toronto, Ontario, Canada).

The National Multiple Sclerosis Society of New York provides many informative and free pamphlets for individuals who have MS, their spouses, significant others, and their children. Topics range from symptoms to sexuality to family emotions.

Local MS organizations or clinics may have additional educational materials, speakers, tapes, etc.

Sick and Tired of Feeling Sick and Tired, P.J. Donoghue, and M.E. Siegle, 1992, New York: W.W. Norton Company.

The MS Autobiography Book, E. Smirnow (ed.), 1992, Cedaredge, Col: Specialized Computer Services.

Three Hundred Tips for Making Life with Multiple Sclerosis Easier, S.P. Schwarz, 1999, New York: Demos.

You Are Not Your Illness: Seven Principles for Meeting the Challenge, L.N. Topf, and H.Z. Bennett, 1995, New York: Simon & Schuster.

Psychosocial Issues in Vocational Success

Significant psychosocial stressors can impact workplace performance or self-advocacy efforts, as noted earlier. Employment rates can be affected by any number of issues: fatigue, visual difficulties, spasticity, coordination issues, or disturbance in bladder and bowel function. These can be problematic for social acceptance reasons on the job as well as because of the practical challenges to performance. Other variables affecting employment outcome are age and educational levels. Workers who are younger or more highly educated fare better in this respect. In addition to societal factors such as discrimination, younger people are more likely to have not progressed as far in the disease process and in related performance difficulties. People with higher educational levels may have better access to mental and physical health care, have skills such as assertiveness, and have other financial and social supports that also improve employment rates.

Cognitive and behavioral changes can further complicate employability. Realistic assessment (of performance difficulties, work site barriers, and compensatory or corrective plans) can prepare the employee for dialogue with his or her employer and reassure the employer. Differentiating social and emotional problems from some neurologically triggered symptoms can be difficult, but is important to successful intervention. Vocational evaluation is discussed in Section III.

Neuropsychological assessment can provide critical information when functional difficulties are disputed (e.g., due to denial, anosagnosia, or simple opinion differences) or when attempts at solutions are significantly frustrated. A six-hour neuropsychological testing battery may be too much for those with MS who fatigue and do not function well at certain times of the day. A neuropsychological assessment that is time-sensitive to a person's current energy level can often assess a person with MS at an optimal functioning level. An argument can also be made for a nonmodified assessment that reflects the true functioning of a person over the course of the work day. If a person can benefit from shift or part-time work, assessing for a time-sensitive optimal functioning profile is very appropriate.

Discrimination has many causes including an ignorance of this complex disease that can leave employers simply bewildered by various MS symptoms and impede helpful accommodation. This may be partially a function of a person with MS being reluctant to address issues due to fear, embarrassment, anosagnosia, denial, or depression. Employers must meet demands for production time lines, work accuracy, and attend to various needs of other workers. They need to be assured that there is a way to keep costs within reason. Most work site accommodations are relatively inexpensive. They often have more to do with flexible and creative problem solving than they do with physical changes to the work site structure or expensive equipment. If physical, cognitive, or emotional symptoms are impacting critical work tasks, a person must disclose their disability and discuss issues with an employer in order to minimize negative reactions at the work site. It is better to start accommodation before the crisis barrel overflows. Clearly proposed solutions and direct negotiation are key. These accommodation strategies should be clarified and addressed, hopefully as part of the initial assessment effort (again see Section III).

It generally is preferable that people with MS present on their own behalf and advocate for themselves effectively. They may need skill building or psychological assistance in preparing to do this for themselves. Because control and loss of control are such large issues with a chronic illness such as MS, the professional should resist the temptation to do more for a worker with MS than that individual can actually do for himself. Successful employer negotiations and experiences will help in overall adjustment and be useful in future nonwork endeavors. An employer is more likely to be less threatened and have a higher regard for an employee who personally can present core performance issues and negotiate a solution than for one who appears to need "rescue" by external rehabilitation consultants. If a person is in acute crisis, has a very passive-dependent personality, or if neurologic changes (sometimes cognitive) make presentation and self-advocacy untenable, scripted written material or alternate representation (i.e., an advocate) may be critical.

Rehearsal before educating or negotiating with an employer is often helpful simply because an employee may be nervous about the employer's reaction or because presentation and negotiation skills need to be cognitively and behaviorally honed. Persons testing out a new job site in which their MS is already known to the employer may encounter and have fewer concerns. A frank discussion about the kinds of adaptations needed in the workplace will help make concerns more understandable and more manageable and will provide for more focused and productive discussion between employer and employee. Those with MS need to be very clear before they have these discussions about: (1) their strengths and deficits, (2) perceived barriers in the workplace, and (3) what they and the employer need to do to compensate for or accommodate these concerns (the Work Experience Survey as discussed in Section III can be very helpful in this process). Presenting in a calm, positive, and nondefensive manner is very important. The presentation should also be clear and as succinct as possible. For example, in relation to memory deficits, "My learning curve is a little slower than some people, but when I learn something it's really hooked in my mind. I'm committed to this job and willing to spend some of my own time memorizing procedures and creating visual memory aids." Interpersonal and audiovisual feedback (viz., video playback) can aid in preparation. Preparation, encouragement, communication, and often back-up written material or "cues" can be helpful. Finding creative solutions requires flexibility on both an employer's and employee's part.

There are many options for accommodation, as reviewed in Section III and within the several illustrations that follow. Knowledge of options can be incredibly empowering. Practical adaptations at a workplace can fail, however, if an individual's emotional and neuro-logic "resistance" to loss and change, or an inordinate stress load, is not adequately addressed. Counseling may need to occur prior to or in tandem with vocational assessment, career transitions review, or work site/style modifications.

A major issue often confronting people with MS and their employers is basic fatigue. They need to sort out the workload for the day so that less demanding tasks can be assigned to that time of the day when fatigue is present. A time-out for a rest, a nap, putting one's feet up either in a car or on a cot in one's office, or an actual break to go home may increase both energy level and mood. The manner in which "off-work time" is to be made up has to be explicit in order to maintain positive work relationships. Employees may need professional assistance in identifying and accepting the manifestations of and accommodations for their fatigue.

An employee may need to prepare a "sales presentation" to an employer in order to convince him or her that working from home is a good idea because, for example, it conserves time and critical energy from commuting to and from work, may allow the person to concentrate more easily when that is a problem, allows the person to take rest breaks thus accommodating health needs, could provide the company early evening business phone contact (if desirable), complies with the ADA inexpensively, and can improve productivity. Workload and supervision time or style may need to be clarified and sometimes redefined. Some weekly time in the office may be required by an employer for work load coordination and staff team building.

Although becoming more mainstream, home-based work reduces community socialization, which may need to be promoted in other ways, particularly when depression and poor self-esteem are present. Working at home can also be distracting. It can lack the structure and familiar cues that some find critical to employment productivity. A realistic assessment of home-based work's validity for an individual or family should be conducted prior to actually submitting a "work at home proposal" to an employer.

Quantifying any decline in production speed or accuracy at a work site or tracing causes can be essential. An employee and employer can then more realistically and positively explore compensatory work product (e.g., work that is taken home to complete after an afternoon rest period has altered the day's productivity). An employee's compensatory efforts allow employers to feel that "they are still getting their money's worth" as they work to accommodate an employee.

Other considerations for an individual with MS may include transportation to and from work, other costs, and possible pay cuts if she has to take a different kind of job that pays less or pays poorly. Those with MS may be less inclined to continue to work if the resulting income is going to be significantly consumed by child care, transportation, and personal aide salaries, and if they perceive that survival would actually be easier if they simply stay home and move to company or federal disability insurance.

An employee with MS may need to address cognitive or emotional changes that impact coworkers, supervision, or task performance. For example, if an employee with MS finds himself or herself being overly chatty, suddenly crying or laughing inappropriately, distracting others, or being more "snappy" with or dependent on others, this individual and the employer may need assistance in planning coping strategies. A coping strategy may need to be concrete, planned, and well-rehearsed. Repetition in using new compensatory behaviors is often important.

Those having difficulties with concentration may need to ask an employer to move them to a place that is less noisy or less socially or visually accessible within the building (to the degree that is possible). A really "chatty" work environment may be especially distracting to people who have concentration or organizational problems. Confronting these problems realistically and finding creative solutions is critical.

External sources of observation and feedback may be helpful to an individual with anasagnosia or memory problems that inhibit self-awareness. This can help open problem-solving discussions. Cognitive problems may necessitate a change of job when deficits are more than can be reasonably accommodated.

Part of a vocational rehabilitation plan may include securing physical, occupational, or speech therapy. Cognitive function compensatory training (e.g., memory/organizational strategies) can often be appropriately provided by speech or occupational therapists. Greater independence can often be maintained and restored through increasing muscle strength and flexibility via physical therapy, hydrotherapy, or yoga. An occupational therapist can be invaluable in assessing and recommending appropriate changes in work activity, tools, or procedures at home sites. (Additional national accommodation resources are referenced in the preceding section.) A psychotherapist can help in overcoming negative resistance, modulating stress, and generally supporting positive efforts.

Successful employment can, as indicated earlier, be dependent on healthy functioning in the social support arena. A person who receives adequate care giving, who doesn't have a "burnt-out" caregiver or spouse at home, and doesn't have distressed children acting out at school or at home is going to function better at work.

Counseling support may be critical for a person to retain meaningful and financially rewarding employment. People may have to struggle to maintain their sense of self-worth relative to the adaptations they need or the type of work that they are able to do if the illness progresses. For example, someone who did a lot of abstract planning may now need to take a less prestigious, more structured, or even supervised job. In this case, a person's self-esteem may be challenged. Depression can increase absenteeism, and decrease productivity or positive relations with others at work. These issues need to be resolved so that a person doesn't sabotage work performance due to conscious or unconscious influences.

Accepting changes such as a need to partially retire early, to no longer be able to drive, and give up other significant elements of independence, can be excruciating. Resistance is likely. This resistance can sometimes threaten the safety and well being of employees, others at the work site, or other drivers on the road. Special counseling that is tailored to a person's age, stage of life, type and level of MS, and grief status can frame a humane intervention that serves worker and community alike.

Considerations in Psychosocial Intervention

Case Study: Mary Jackson

Ms. Jackson is not a real person, but her case illustrates a number of the issues that have been presented to the author during her career in social services or social services administration for those with MS.

Identifying Information

Mary Jackson was diagnosed with MS three years ago. She is 39 years old, recently separated from her husband of 14 years, and has two children ages 6 and 13. She is neatly dressed, has a coffee and cream complexion, hazel eyes, tight curly hair, and is "about 40 pounds overweight" (gained since her diagnosis). She says her mother is German and her father is Irish/African-American.

Employment Status

Mary has lost her job as a sale representative for the All Service Computer Company because she cannot travel, be on her feet, nor handle the high energy demands of her sales job. She performed well and was highly regarded by her company. She declined the one alternative job option offered by the company, that of secretary. She says that several prospective employers have seemed to react negatively to her balance and speech problems in the actual interview or post-interview, repeatedly asking questions about her "recreational" activities and seeming to suspect alcohol or drug use.

Social Status

Her husband has "begun to drink," she says, and the oldest girl has been acting out at school these past five weeks. Mary describes her husband, Roger, as a hard-working engineer, a farmer's son, who cannot tolerate the changes in their lifestyle (e.g., her declining housework, reduced sexual activity) due to her fatigue. The couple are currently separated with Roger living out of the home. She has no other close family, and few close friends.

Physical Status

She has had intermittent MS physical symptoms for the last six years. All exacerbations have been followed by full remission except the last two, which have left her with profound afternoon fatigue and with minor balance and slurred speech difficulties. Optic neuritis occurs occasionally with her exacerbations.

Cognitive Status

During periods of fatigue Mary experiences sluggish "multitasking" abilities, reduced information processing speed, and poor short-term verbal memory.

Emotional Status

She sits rigidly and smiles a strained smile in the initial interview. Mary reports difficulty modifying her energy expenditure in order to accommodate periods of fatigue and expresses great frustration and intolerance for her physical and cognitive changes. She is anxious that her husband may not return or support the family and that she may not be able "make ends meet." She is distressed and distracted about her daughter's reactions to her MS and the marital separation.

Issues in the Case of Mary

Questions:

- What are the psychosocial issues that the client needs to deal with for successful employment?
- What challenges might this employee and an employer have to deal with to better meet everyone's needs?
- How can you best assist this client (goals and objectives)?

Considerations:

- What resources might be accessed (evaluative, support, education, mentoring, etc.) to best serve this client?
- How and when will you pursue these resources?
- Are there issues you are choosing to not address?
- Why might you choose not to address them and is there any potential impact to not addressing them?

Discussion: Intervention Considerations in the Case of Mary

It would be important to secure a release from Ms. Jackson and pursue information from her primary care physician and neurologist about her level of function, MS exacerbations, and prognosis. This could also help to establish a differential diagnosis between disease versus emotionally based cognitive impairment. Some testing or evaluation of her cognitive function could be helpful to establishing the nature of an employment position or job site accommodations that would now be appropriate. It would also be helpful to know if there are some medications or other medical interventions that have been tried or will be tried and, if they have been tried, and to what degree of success for this particular individual (e.g., for the fatigue concern).

Referral to State Vocational Rehabilitation, often through an area Project with Industry placement program or an MS organization, can be critical to support the cost of vocational evaluation, neuropsychological assessment, assistive technology consultation (for potential job site accommodations, etc.), diverse medical consultation, and other services.

Allied health services can help to round out needed services. Speech therapy may help her with her slurred speech difficulty. A medical assessment for potential optic neuritis intervention could be helpful. Are there compensatory interventions that could be utilized? Issues related to sexual functioning may need to be reviewed for Mary (and perhaps her husband) at a specialty clinic. Physical therapy could help her with balance training. Speech therapy could also help her with memory and organizational aids and address her cognitive functioning problems in order to improve her social and later job functioning. Occupational therapists can also be very helpful with cognitive compensatory strategies and rehearsal.

Family counseling that is informational and supportive could help Mary, her daughters, and hopefully her husband sort out their various MS-related concerns. As she confronts significant others clearly, she may clarify what allies she really has within this adjustment period.

Mary will need specialized personal counseling, ideally of a cognitive-behavioral nature, that "fits" within the psychotherapy framework usually supported by the State Rehabilitation Agency—often 10 to 12 sessions to assist in "jump-starting" proactive adjustment efforts. The focus might be on coping and problem solving strategies in dealing with her family members. Coping strategies to handle her own anxiety and depression would be very important. Grief support could be provided in tandem.

Since she has limited family, few close friends, and a "questionable" husband, she is also in need of social support beyond just the professional. She may want to connect with a woman's group, one-to-one peer support, telephone support, or an MS Internet support or chat group. She simply needs to expand her social support system. She could address the issue of mustering social support within her personal counseling sessions.

Another consideration of course is that she is dealing with not only having to sell herself as a woman to employers, but also as a person of color with a disability. She has three separate challenges here, and she can benefit from support and assistance in how to handle them. She clearly has a skill base and has made it over a number of vocational hurdles already. Perhaps the skill base can be retooled and reaffirmed, but clearly she does need some support.

She needs an immediate plan for her core financial security (considering potential federal or other subsidy). Knowing that there's a safety net for the family's essentials can free up emotional energy needed further up the hierarchy of needs. Because Mary does appear rather proud, a respectful and empowering approach will be especially important to her. You want to support her strengths, dignity, and self-control and at the same time offer her options to support herself in ways that allow her to see that she is taking steps to regain control of her life.

Summary

Multiple sclerosis is a varied and unpredictable disease that can usher in a host of major and minor symptoms that are physical, cognitive, or emotional. This disease impacts not only the person who has the disease, but the whole family and related support systems. A systems perspective is needed to intervene adequately.

The individual and his family may need information, supportive emotional counseling, and practical cognitive-behavioral approaches that encourage engagement rather than long-term insight-oriented therapy. There is a need for individual, but also often family or group counseling, involvement. Spouses, significant others, and children are often underserved, and tend to remain "invisible" as services are provided to the person who has MS. Significant others as caregivers can profit from counseling and training regarding balance of personal needs in their lives. It is very natural and normal for an individual and his family to have a grief reaction that can include sadness or depression, anxiety, shock, denial, and so forth. Feelings of despair or suicidal thinking can occur as a part of the grief reaction.

Employers often need practical information and creative problem solving assistance to accommodate an individual with these disabilities. Assisting the individual with MS to learn or enhance skills in self advocacy can improve vocational outlook and empower the client in other arenas as well.

A service plan should be tailored to a specific individual's physical and cognitive symptoms, emotional responses, and resources within their support systems. Because the disability is so variable, it is important to not generalize about MS or reactions to MS.

It is critical that the individual and his family have adequate support and information from the health sciences community (e.g., physical therapy, occupational therapy, speech and language therapy), and that the psychotherapy and medical professionals are working as a team and communicating. The individual and his family or significant other may need not only information about the disease and relevant interventions, but how to maintain viable living situations and relationships.

The author wishes you well in your work in this arena and thanks you for your compassionate efforts on behalf of individuals and families living with MS.

References

Barak, Y., Achrion, A., Elizur, A., Gabbay, U., and Noy, S. (1996). Sexual dysfunction in relapsing-remitting multiple sclerosis: Magnetic resonance imaging, clinical and psychological correlates. *J Psychiatry Neurosci* 21(4):255–258.

Baumgarten, M., Hanley, J.A., and Infante-Rivard, C. et al. (1994). Health of family members caring for elderly persons with dementia. *Ann Intern Med* 120:126–132.

Braham, S., Houser, H.B., and Cline, A. et al. (1975). Evaluation of the social needs of nonhospitalized chronically ill persons: Study of 47 patients with multiple sclerosis. *J Chronic Dis* 28:401–419.

Brooks, N.A., and Matson, R. (1987). Managing multiple sclerosis. *Res Sociol Health Care* 6:73–106.

Burnfield, A., and Burnfield, P. (1982). Common psychological problems in multiple sclerosis. *Br Med J*, 1:1193–1194.

Carroll, D.L., and Dorman, J.D. (1993). *Living well with MS: A guide for patient, caregiver, and family*. New York: HarperCollins.

Foley, F.W., Sexuality and Intimacy in Multiple Sclerosis, in *Multuiple Sclerosis: A Guide for Families*, Rosalind C. Kalb, Ph.D., ed., New York: Demos, 1998.

Frankel, D., and Buxbuam, R. (1982). Maximizing your health. Massachusetts chapter: National MS Society.

Kalb, R.C. (1998). *Multiple sclerosis: A guide for families*. New York: Demos.

Kraft, G., and Catanzaro, M. (second edition 1999). *Living with multiple sclerosis: A wellness approach*. New York: Demos.

Kroll, K., and Klein, E.L. (1992). *Enabling romance: A guide to love, sex, and relationships for the disabled*. New York: Harmony Books.

LeMaistre, J. (1985). *Beyond rage*. Oak Park, Ill.: Alpine Guild (also in audio).

LeMaistre, J. (1995). *After the diagnosis*. Berkeley, Calif.: Ulysses Press.

Luterman, D. (1995). In the shadows: *Living and coping with a loved one's chronic illness*. Bedford, Mass.: Jade Press.

Maurer, J.R., and Strasberg,P.D. (1990). *Building a new dream—A family guide to coping with chronic illness and disability*. New York: Addison-Wesley Publishing Company, Inc.

Minden, S.L., and Frankel, D. (1987; revised 1992). *Plaintalk. A booklet about multiple sclerosis for family members*. New York: National MS Society.

Murray, T.J. (1995). The psychosocial aspects of multiple sclerosis. *Neurol Clin Fed* 13(1):197–223.

Neistadt, M.E., and Feda, M. (1987). *Choices: A guide to sex counseling with physically disabled adults*. Malabar, Fla.: Robert E. Krieger Publishing.

Ottenberg, M. (1978). *Pursuit of hope*. New York: Rawson Wade, Inc.

Provinciali, L., Ceravolo, M.D., Batolini, M., Logutto, F., and Danni, M. (1999). A multidimensional assessment of multiple sclerosis: Relationship between disability domains. *Acta Neurol Scand* 100(3):156–162.

Rao, S.M. (1986). Neuropsychology of multiple sclerosis: A critical review. *J Clin Exp Neuropsych* 8:503–546.

Ritvo, P.G., Fisk, J.D., and Archibald, C.J. et al. (1992). A model of mental health in patients with multiple sclerosis. *Can Psychol* 33:391.

Rosner, L.J. (1987). *Multiple sclerosis: New hope and practical advice for people with MS and their families*. New York: Prentice Hall.

Rumrill, P. (1997). *Employment issues and multiple sclerosis*. New York: Demos.

Simons, A.F. (1984). *Multiple sclerosis: Psychological and social aspects*. London: William Heinemann Medical Books.

Strong, Maggie. (1989). *Mainstay*. New York: Penguin Books.

APPENDIX A

U.S. Department of Labor
Employment Standards Administration
Wage and Hour Division
Washington, DC 20210

Statement of Principle

The U.S. Department of Labor and community-based rehabilitation organizations are committed to the continued development and implementation of individual vocational rehabilitation programs that will facilitate the transition of persons with disabilities into employment within their communities. This transition must take place under conditions that will not jeopardize the protections afforded by the Fair Labor Standards Act to program participants, employees, employers, or other programs providing rehabilitation services to individuals with disabilities.

Guidelines

Where ALL of the following criteria are met, the U.S. Department of Labor will NOT assert an employment relationship for purposes of the Fair Labor Standards Act.

- Participants will be individuals with physical and/or mental disabilities for whom competitive employment at or above the minimum wage level is not immediately obtainable and who, because of their disability, will need intensive ongoing support to perform in a work setting.
- Participation will be for vocational exploration, assessment or training in a community-based placement work site under the general supervision of rehabilitation organization personnel.
- Community-based placement will be clearly defined components of individual rehabilitation programs developed and designed for the benefit of each individual. The statement of needed transition services established for the exploration, assessment or training components will be included in the person's Individualized Written Rehabilitation Plan (IWRP).
- Information obtained in the IWRP will not have to be made available, however; documentation as to the individual's enrollment in the community-based placement program will be made available to the Department of Labor. The individual and, when appropriate, the parent or guardian of each individual, must be fully informed of the IWRP and the community-based placement component and have indicated voluntary participation with the understanding that participation in such a component does not entitle the participant to wages.
- The activities of the individuals at the community-based placement site does not result in an immediate advantage to the business. The Department of Labor will look at several factors.

1. There has been no displacement of employees, vacant positions have not been filled, employees have not been relieved of assigned duties, and the individuals are not performing services that, although not ordinarily performed by employees, clearly are of benefit to the business.

2. The individuals are under continued and direct supervision by either representatives of the rehabilitation facility or by employees of the business.

3. Such placements are made according to the requirements of the individual's IWRP and not to meet the labor needs of the business.

4. The periods of time spent by the individuals at any one site or in any clearly distinguishable job classification are specifically limited by the IWRP.

- While the existence of an employment relationship will not be determined exclusively on the basis of the number of hours, as a general rule, each component will not exceed the following limitations:

Vocational explorations	5 hours per job experienced
Vocational assessment	90 hours per job experienced
Vocational training	120 hours per job experienced

An employment relationship will exist unless *all of the criteria* described in the policy are met. If an employment relationship is found to exist, the business will be held responsible for full compliance with the applicable sections of the Fair Labor Standards Act, including those relating to child labor.

Businesses and rehabilitation organizations may, at any time, consider participants to be employees and may structure the program so that the participants are compensated in accordance with the requirements of the Fair Labor Standards Act. Whenever an employment relationship is established, the business may make use of the special minimum wage provisions provided pursuant to section 14(c) of the Act.

Donald J. Hinkel, Chair
National Rehabilitation Facilities Coalition

Karen R. Keesling, Acting Administrator
Wage and Hour Division
U.S. Department of Labor

Work Experience Survey

Note: Appreciation is extended to Dr. Richard Roessler and the Arkansas Research and Training Center staff for the use of this instrument—all users of the instrument need to maintain the page referencing Dr. Roessler and the Arkansas Research and Training Center.

WORK EXPERIENCE SURVEY (WES)

Section I: Please provide information on your background, disability, and work experience.

Background

1. Age_____   2. Sex_____   3. Race_____   4. Marital status_____
5. Number of years of education_____
6. Highest educational degree completed_____

Disability

7. Disability of record (primary diagnosis)_____
8. How old were you when you acquired this disability?_____
9. What caused your disability?_____
10. Describe how the disability affects your functioning, e.g., decrease in muscle strength, chronic fatigue, limited visual field, poor balance, low stress tolerance. Rank order the entries in terms of their impact, e.g., the first effect listed represents the greatest problem.
    1. _____
    2. _____
    3. _____
    4. _____
    5. _____

Work Experience

11. You current job title (the one used by your employer)_____
12. List three essential job functions that you perform regularly, e.g., take telephone messages, operate forklift, feed/care for livestock.
    _____
    _____
    _____

13. Name/address of company where you work_____
    Street Address:_____
    City_____ State_____ Zip code_____
14. Total number of years employed_____
15. Number of months on current job_____
16. Number of hours working per week_____
17. Weekly gross salary_____

Section II: Accessibility: Check (✔) any problems you have getting
to, from, or around on your job. List any other accessibility problems
not included in the list. Describe solutions for your two most important accessibility barriers.

___Parking   ___Bathrooms   ___Temperature
___Public walks   ___Water fountains   ___Ventilation
___Passenger loading zones   ___Public telephone   ___Hazards
___Entrance   ___Elevators   ___Identification signs/labels
___Stairs/Steps   ___Lighting   ___Access to personnel offices
___Floors/Floor covering   ___Warning devices   ___Access to general use areas
___Seating/Tables   ___Evacuation routes

List any other accessibility problems:
#1_____

_____
#2_____

_____

Describe solutions for your two most important accessibility barriers.
#1_____

_____
#2_____

_____

Section III: Essential job functions: Check (✔) any essential job functions or conditions* that pose problems for you. Describe the two most important job modifications that you need, e.g., modifying existing equipment, adding new technology, or changing the type of work you do.

Physical Abilities

___Working 8 hours

___Standing all day

___Standing part of the time

___Walking for 8 hours

___Some kneeling

___Some stooping

___Some climbing

___Much pulling

___Much pushing

___Much talking

___Seeing well

___Hearing well

___Handling

___Raising arms above
    shoulders

___Using both hands

___Using both legs

___Using left hand

___Using right hand

___Using left leg

___Using right leg

___Lifting over 100 lbs.

___Lifting 51–100 lbs.

___Lifting 26–50 lbs.

___Lifting 11–25 lbs.

___Lifting 0–10 lbs.

___Prolonged sitting

Cognitive Abilities

___Immediate memory

___Short-term memory

___Long-term memory

___Judgment: safety

___Judgment: interpersonal

___Thought processing

___Reasoning

___Problem solving

___Planning

___Organizing

Task Related Abilities

___Repetitive work

___Work pace/sequenacing

___Variety of duties

___Perform under stress/
    deadlines

___little feedback on performance

___Read written instructions

___Able and licensed to drive

___Attain precise standards/limits

___Follow specific instructions

___Writing

___Remembering

___Speaking/Communicating

___Initiating work activities

___Use telephone

Social Abilities

___Working alone

___Working around others

___Working with others

___Interacting with supervisors

___Supervising others

___Working with hostile others

Working Conditions

___Too hot

___Too cold

___Temperature changes

___Too wet

___Too humid

___Slippery surfaces

___Obstacles in path

___Dust

___Fumes

___Odors

___Noise

___Outdoors

___Sometimes outdoors

___Always inside

Company Policies

___Inflexible work schedules

___No accrual of sick lease

___Lack of flextime

___No "comp" time

___Inflexible job descriptions

___Vague job descriptions

___Infrequent reviews of job
    descriptions

___Rigid sick/vacation leave policies

*Adapted from *RehabMatch*. Arkansas Research and Training Center in Vocational Rehabilitation.

Describe the two job modifications that would be most helpful to you, e.g., restructuring of the job, modification of work schedules, reassignment to another position, modification of equipment, or provision of readers and interpreters.

#1_____

_____

#2_____

_____

Section IV: Job Mastery: Check (✔) any concerns* that affect your success in completing the following tasks. Describe one solution for each of your two most important concerns.

1. Getting the job done
    ___Believing that others think I do a good job.
    ___Understanding how my job fits into the "big picture," i.e., the meaning of my job.
    ___Knowing what I need to know to do my job.
    ___Having what I need to do my job (knowledge, tools, supplies, equipment).
2. Fitting into the workforce
    ___Scheduling and planning my work ahead of time.
    ___Working mostly because I like the job.
    ___Doing a good job.
    ___Willing to make changes when necessary.
3. Learning the ropes
    ___Knowing who to go to if I need help.
    ___Understanding company rules and regulations.
    ___Knowing my way around work.
    ___Feeling a "part" of what is going on at work.
4. Getting along with others
    ___Eating lunch with friends at work.
    ___Having many friends at work.

---

*Selected items from the Career Mastery Inventory. Used with permission of the author, John O. Crites, Crites Career Consultants, Boulder, Colorado.

___Looking forward to seeing my friends at work.

___Knowing what is expected of me socially on the job.

5. Getting ahead

___Having a plan for where I want to be in my job in the future.

___Understanding what I have to do to get promoted.

___Knowing what training to complete to improve chances for promotion.

___Talking with supervisor about what I need to do to get promoted.

6. Planning the next career step

___Considering what I will do in the future.

___Knowing what the opportunities are in this company.

___Wanting to become more specialized in my job.

___Having a good idea of how to advance in this company.

Describe one solution for each of your two most important job mastery concerns.

#1_____

_____

#2_____

_____

Section V. Satisfaction*: Rate your current job on each of the following statements. Describe two ways to make your job more personally satisfying.

In my job ... (check one)	Too Little	About Right	Too Much
I do things that make use of my abilities.	__	__	__
The job gives me a feeling of accomplishment.	__	__	__
I am busy all the time.	__	__	__
I can work alone on the job.	__	__	__
I do something different every day.	__	__	__

*Work reinforcers from the Minnesota Theory of Work Adjustment. Dawis, R. & Lofquist, L. (1984). A psychological theory of work adjustment. Minneapolis: University of Minnesota.

In my job ... (check one)	Too Little	About Right	Too Much
My pay compares well with that of other workers.	—	—	—
The job provides for steady employment.	—	—	—
The job has good working conditions.	—	—	—
The job provides an opportunity for advancement.	—	—	—
I get recognition for the work I do.	—	—	—
I tell people what to do.	—	—	—
I am "somebody" in the community.	—	—	—
My co-workers are easy to make friends with.	—	—	—
I can do the work without feeling it is morally wrong.	—	—	—
I can do things for other people.	—	—	—
The company administers its policies fairly.	—	—	—
My boss backs up the workers with top management.	—	—	—
My boss trains the workers well.	—	—	—
I try out some of my ideas.	—	—	—
I make decisions on my own.	—	—	—

Describe two ways to make your job more personally satisfying.

#1_____

_____

#2_____

_____

Section VI. Review Sections II-V of the WES and list the three most significant barriers to success in your work. Describe their solutions and people/resources who can help. Be specific.

Barrier 1:_____

    Solution?_____

    _____

    _____

    _____

    Who can help? How can they help?_____

    _____

    _____

    _____

Barrier 2:_____

    Solution?_____

    _____

    _____

    _____

    Who can help? How can they help?_____

    _____

    _____

    _____

Barrier 3:_____

    Solution?_____

    _____

    _____

    _____

    Who can help? How can they help?_____

    _____

    _____

    _____

MS Information Treatment Centers

The following clinical facilities have a formal affiliation with the National Multiple Sclerosis Society. The appropriate chapter clinical advisory committee, composed of MS experts, has reviewed and approved the affiliation.

Alabama

Neurology Department, UAB
The School of Medicine
University of Alabama
University Station
Birmingham, AL 35294
(205) 934-2402

California

Neurology Medical Group of
    Diablo Valley, Inc.
130 La Casa Via, #206
Walnut Creek, CA 94598
(510) 939-9400

1844 San Miguel Drive, #316
Walnut Creek, CA 94596
(510) 938-5252

Parnassus MS Center
900 Parnassus Ave
San Francisco, CA 94117
(415) 476-4173

St. Mary's Hospital, MS Clinic
2200 Hayes St.
San Francisco, CA 94117
(415) 750-5762

Mount Zion MS Center, UCSF
1600 Divisadero St.
San Francisco, CA 94115
(415) 885-7844

East Bay Neurology
3000 Colby St., #201
Berkeley, CA 94705
(510) 849-0159

University of California
107 Irvine Hall
Irvine, CA 92717
(714) 824-5692

Department of Rehabilitation, MS
    Clinic
Santa Clara Valley Medical Center
751 S. Bascom Avenue
San Jose, CA 95128
(408) 885-2000 (408) 885-2028

Kaiser-Permanente Medical Center
900 Keily Blvd.
Santa Clara, CA 95051
(408) 236-4999

Transitions Rehabilitation MS
    Clinic
7101 Monterey Street, Suite A
Gilroy, CA 95020
(408) 842-6868

Reed Neurological Research Center,
    UCLA
PO Box 951769
Los Angeles, CA 90095-1769
(310) 825-7313 (310) 206-9801

UCLA-Neurological Services
300 Medical Plaza, Suite B200
Los Angeles, CA 90024-6975
(310) 794-1195 (310) 794-7491 (FAX)

MS Comprehensive Care Center at
    USC University Hospital
1510 San Pablo Street, Sixth Floor
Los Angeles, CA 90033-4606
(323) 442-6870 (323) 442-5773 (FAX)

Cedars Sinai Medical Center, MS
  Treatment Center
8631 W. 3rd Street, 1001 E Tower
Los Angeles, CA 90048
(310) 855-6472 (310) 967-0130 (FAX)

Harbor-UCLA Medical Center, MS
  Clinic
1000 W. Carson Street
Torrance, CA 90505
(310) 322-3897 (310) 533-8905 (FAX)

Rancho Los Amigos Hospital
Division of Neurosciences
7601 E. Imperial Way
Building #800, Annex West
Downey, CA 90242
(562) 401-7713 or (562) 401-7093
(562) 401-6247 (FAX)

Connecticut

Gaylord Hospital MS Clinic
PO Box 400
Wallingford, CT 06492
(203) 284-2845

Yale University School of Medicine
  MS Clinic
40 Temple Street, Suite 71
New Haven, CT 06510-8018
(203) 764-4280

West Haven–VAMC
Multiple Sclerosis Program
950 Campbell Avenue
West Haven, CT 06516
(203) 937-4735

Florida

North Florida MS Comprehensive
  Care Center at St. Luke's
  Hospital
4203 Belfort Road
Rodget Main Building, Suite 115
Jacksonville, FL 32216
(904) 296-5731 (904) 296-4088 (FAX)

Healthsouth Sea Pine
  Rehabilitation Hospital
101 E. Florida Avenue
Melbourne, FL 32901
(407) 984-4600

MS Clinic
Healthsouth Rehabilitation
3251 Proctor Road
Sarasota, FL 34231
(941) 921-8600

Neurological Center
12901 Bruce B. Downs Avenue
Tampa, FL 33612
(813) 974-2722

Baptist Medical Art Building—MS
  Clinic
8940 N. Kendall Drive, Suite 802E
Miami, FL 33176
(305) 596-4041

Georgia

St. Joseph's Hospital MS Clinic
Chandler Heart & Lung Bldg.
5356 Reynolds Street, Suite 200
Savannah, GA 31405
(800) 921-3212

Shepherd Center, Inc.
2020 Peachtree Road NW
Atlanta, GA 30309
(404) 350-7392

DeKalb Medical Center
2675 N. Decatur Road, Suite 105
Decatur, GA 30033
(404) 501-5140

Illinois

Loyola University Medical Center
    MS Clinic
2160 S. 1st Avenue
Maywood, IL 60153
(708) 216-6001

Pritzker University Medical Center
    MS Clinic
University of Chicago
Department of Neurology
5841 S. Maryland Avenue
Chicago, IL 60637
(312) 702-6386

1725 W. Harrison Street, Suite 309
Chicago, IL 60612
(312) 942-8011

Northwestern University
Department of Neurology
Medical School, Suite 500
233 E. Erie Street
Chicago, IL 60611
(312) 908-7950

214 North East Glen Oak Avenue
Peoria, IL 61603
(309) 676-2616

Southern Illinois University
School of Medicine
Department of Neurology
Baylis Medical Building
747 N. Rutlidge
Springfield, IL 62781
(217) 788-3391

Indiana

Caylor-Nickel Comprehensive MS
    Clinic
One Caylor-Nickel Square
Bluffton, IN 46714
(219) 824-3500

Indiana University MS Center
550 North University Blvd., Rm.
    1719
Indianapolis, IN 46202-5111
(317) 278-2771

Indiana Center for MS and
    Neuroimmunopathologic and
    Disorders
8424 Noah Road, #1A
Indianapolis, IN 46260
(317) 614-3100

Kentucky

University of Kentucky
Chandler Medical Center
Department of Neurology
Kentucky Clinic, L445
Lexington, KY 40536-0284
(606) 323-6702

University of Louisville
Department of Neurology
601 S. Floyd Street, #503
Louisville, KY 40202
(606) 258-6830 (606) 258-6840 (FAX)

Frazier Rehabilitation Center
220 Abraham Flexner Way
Louisville, KY 40202-1887
(502) 582-7400

Baptist Hospital East, Neuroscience
  Associates
6400 Dutchmans Parkway, Suite
  140
Louisville, KY 40205
(502) 895-7265

Purchase Area MS Clinic
225 Medical Center Drive, Suite 402
Paducah, KY 42002-8129
(502) 441-4400

Louisiana

MS Clinic, Neurology Clinic
Tulane Medical Center
1415 Tulane Avenue
New Orleans, LA 70112
(504) 588-5231

Maine

Maine Neurology, P.A.
49 Spring Street
Scarborough, ME 04074
(207) 883-1414

Maryland

University of Maryland
Department of Neurology
The School of Medicine
22 S. Greene Street
Baltimore, MD 21201
(410) 328-5605

Johns Hopkins Hospital
Department of Neurology
600 N. Wolfe Street, Meyer 6-113
Baltimore, MD 21287-7613
(410) 955-5103

Union Memorial Hospital
3333 N. Calvert Street, Suite 300
Baltimore, MD 21218
(410) 554-2318

Massachusetts

Mount Auburn Hospital
300 Mt Auburn Street, Suite 316
Cambridge, MA 02138
(617) 868-5014

Metro West Medical Center
115 Lincoln Street
Framingham, MA 07101
(508) 879-1911

Michigan

Wayne State University
The School of Medicine
Department of Neurology
University Health Center, 6E
4201 St. Antoine
Detroit, MI 48201
(313) 745-4275 (313) 745-4468 (FAX)

Michigan State University
138 Service Road
A-217 Clinical Center
East Lansing, MI 48824
(517) 353-8122 (517) 432-3713 (FAX)

Henry Ford Hospital
Department of Neurology
2799 W. Grand Blvd.
Detroit, MI 48202
(313) 876-7207 (313) 876-3014 (FAX)

Mid-Michigan Regional Medical
   Center
4011 Orchard Drive, Suite 4010
Midland, MI 48640
(517) 835-8744 (517) 839-3369 (FAX)

Minnesota
Fairview MS Center
Riverside Park Plaza
701 25th Avenue South, #200
Minneapolis, MN 55454
(612) 672-6100

St. Mary's/Duluth Clinic
Health System
400 E. 3rd Street
Duluth, MN 55805
(218) 725-3925

Missouri
Washington University MS Clinic
School of Medicine
Department of Neurology
Box 8111
660 S. Euclid
St. Louis, MO 63110
(314) 362-3293

Nebraska
University of Medical Associates at
   the University of Nebraska
   Medical Clinic
600 S. 42nd Street
Omaha, NE 68198
(402) 559-7859

Nevada
50 Kirman Avenue, #201
Reno, NV 89502
(775) 324-2234 (775) 324-6015

New Jersey
Gimbel MS Center
718 Teaneck Road
Teaneck, NJ 07666
(201) 837-0727 (201) 837-8503 (FAX)

RM Research and Treatment
   Center of UMDNY
185 S. Orange Avenue, H506
Newark, NJ 07103
(201) 982-2550

New Mexico
University of Mexico
Department of Neurology
1201 Yale Blvd. NE
Albuquerque, NM 87131
(505) 272-3342 (505) 272-4056 (FAX)

New York
MS Care Center at Mercy Medical
   Center Physical Therapy Center
128 Atlantic Avenue
Lynbrook, NY 11563
(516) 596-0700

SUNY at Sony Brook
Department of Neurology
Health Science Center, T-12, Room
  020
Stony Brook, NY 11790
(516) 444-1450

South Shore Neurologic Associates,
  PC
877 E. Main Street
Riverhead, NY 11901
(516) 727-0660

Care Center at North Shore
  University Hospital at Sysosset
221 Jericho Turnpike
Syosset, NY 11791
(516) 727-0660

Maimonides Medical Center
4802 Tenth Avenue
Brooklyn, NY 11219
(718) 283-7470

Columbia-Presbyterian Medical
  Center
MS Care Center
Vanderbilt Clinic
710 W. 168th Street
New York, NY 10032
(212) 305-5508

Columbia-Presbyterian Medical
  Center
MS Care Center
16 E. 60th Street
New York, NY 10022
(212) 326-8455

NY Hospital Medical Center
Queens MS Care Center
Department of Neurology
56-45 Main Street
Flushing, NY 11355
(718) 460-6765 or (718) 460-2903

The New York Hospital–Cornell
  Medical Center
525 E. 68th Street
New York, NY 10021
(212) 746-4504

Staten Island University Hospital
Irving R. Boody Jr. Medical Arts
  Pavilion
475 Seaview Avenue
Staten Island, NY 10305
(718) 667-3800

Bronx-Lebanon Hospital
1770 Grand Concourse
Bronx, NY 10457
(718) 960-1335

Hospital for Joint Diseases
301 E. 17th Street
New York, NY 10003
(212) 598-6305

St. Luke's-Roosevelt Medical
  Center
MS Treatment & Research Center
425 W. 59th Street, Suite 7C
New York, NY 10019
(212) 523-8070

Strong Memorial Hospital
University of Rochester
601 Elmwood Avenue
Rochester, NY 14642-8873
(716) 275-7854 (716) 442-9480 (FAX)

Helen Hayes Hospital MS Clinic
Route 9W
West Haverstraw, NY 10993
(914) 947-3000

William C. Baird MS Research
    Center
Millard Fillmore Hospital
3 Gates Circle
Buffalo, NY 14209
(716) 887-5230 (716) 887-4285 (FAX)

St. Agnes MS Center
303 North Street, Suite 203
White Plains, NY 10605
(914) 328-6410

Buffalo General Hospital
100 High Street
Buffalo, NY 14203
(716) 859-7592 (716) 859-2430 (FAX)

North Carolina
MS Center at Carolinas Medical
    Center
PO Box 32861
Charlotte, NC 28232-2861
(704) 342-7300

Ohio
Mellen Center U-10
Cleveland Clinic Foundation
9500 Euclid Avenue
Cleveland, OH 44195
(216) 445-6800

Ohio State University Medical Center
Department of Neurology
466 W. 10th Avenue
Columbus, OH 43210-1228
(614) 293-4964 (614) 293-6111

Oregon
OHSU MS Clinic
Department of Neurology, L 226
Oregon Health Science University
3181 South West Sam Jackson Park
    Road
Portland, OR 97201
(503) 494-5759 (503) 494-7242 (FAX)

Pennsylvania
University of Pittsburgh
811 Lillian Kaufman Building
3471 Fifth Avenue
Pittsburgh, PA 15213
(412) 692-4915 (412) 692-4907 (FAX)

Allegheny University MS
    Treatment Center
420 East North Avenue, Suite 206
Pittsburgh, PA 15212
(412) 321-2162 (412) 321-5073 (FAX)

The College of Medicine
Pennsylvania State University
500 University Drive
Hershey, PA 17033
(717) 531-8692 (717) 531-4694 (FAX)

Geisinger Clinic, 14-05
100 North Academy Avenue
Danville, PA 17822-1405
(717) 271-6590

Lehigh Valley Hospital
Neuroscience Research
1243 S. Cedar Crest Blvd.,
    Suite 3232
Allentown, PA 18103
(610) 403-9330

MCP Hahnemann University
3300 Henry Avenue
Philadelphia, PA 19129
(215) 842-7717

Hospital of the University of
    Pennsylvania
3 West Gates Building
3400 Spruce Street
Philadelphia, PA 19104-4283
(215) 662-6565

Reading Rehabilitation Hospital
    MS Clinic
1623 Morgantown Road
Reading, PA 19607-4555
(610) 796-6000

Thomas Jefferson University
    Hospital
Neurology Department
835 Chestnut Street, 4th Floor
Philadelphia, PA 19107
(215) 955-6692

Temple University Hospital
Department of Neurology
3400 N. Broad Street
Philadelphia, PA 19140
(215) 221-3040

South Carolina
Medical University at SC
171 Ashley Avenue
Charleston, SC 29425
(843) 792-3221 (843) 792-8626 (FAX)

Texas
Baylor Methodist International MS
    Center
6560 Fannin, Suite 1224
Houston, TX 77030
(713) 798-7707

Ben Taub Hospital MS Clinic
1504 Taub Loop
Houston, TX 77030

Utah
The School of Medicine
University of Utah
50 North Medical Drive
Salt Lake City, UT 84132
(801) 585-6032 or (801) 581-4283

Vermont
Fletcher Allen Health Care
Multiple Sclerosis Clinic
FAHC-UHC Campus
1 South Prospect Street
Burlington, VT 05401
(802) 656-4589

Virginia
DePaul Medical Center MS Clinic
6161 Kemsville Circle, #315
Norfolk, VA 23505
(757) 461-5400 or (757) 889-5201

Washington
Multiple Sclerosis Clinic
Overlake Hospital
1035 116th Avenue NE
Bellevue, WA 98004
(425) 688-5900 (425) 688-5912 (FAX)

Multiple Sclerosis Clinic
The School of Medicine
University of Washington
BB933 Health Sciences Bldg. (Box
    356490)
Seattle, WA 98195-6490
(206) 543-7272 (206) 685-3244 (FAX)

Holy Family Hospital MS Center
5901 N. Lidgerwood, Suite 25B
Spokane, WA 99207
(509) 489-5019

Wisconsin
The Marshfield Clinic, MS Clinic
1000 North Oak Avenue
Marshfield, WI 54449
(715) 387-9115

Medical College of Wisconsin
Department of Neurology
Clinic at Froedtert
9200 W. Wisconsin Avenue
Milwaukee, WI 53226
(414) 454-5200

University of Wisconsin
Department of Neurology
Medical School
600 Highland Avenue
Madison, WI 53792
(608) 263-5448

Center for Neurological Disorders
St. Francis Hospital
3237 South 16th Street
Milwaukee, WI 53215
(414) 647-5305

National Multiple Sclerosis Society Chapters/Divisions/Branches

Note: * indicates affiliate with strong vocational component—see Colorado chapter for National Employment Resource.

Alabama

Alabama Chapter
3530 Independence Drive, Suite 3534
Birmingham, AL 35209
(205) 879-8881

Alaska

Alaska Division
511 W. 41st Ave., Suite 11
Anchorage, AK 99503
(907) 563-1115

Arizona

Desert Southwest Chapter/Phoenix
    Branch
315 S. 48th St., #101
Tempe, AZ 85281
(480) 968-2488

Tucson Branch/Desert Southwest
    Chapter
626 N. Craycroft, Suite 116
Tucson, AZ 85711
(520) 747-7472

Arkansas

Arkansas Division
Evergreen Place
1100 N. University, Suite 255
Little Rock, AR 72207
(501) 663-6767

California

Channel Islands Chapter
14 W. Valerio St
Santa Barbara, CA 93101
(805) 682-8783

Mountain Valley California Chapter
2277 Watt Ave., Suite 300
Sacramento, CA 95825
(916) 427-3310

Northern California Chapter
150 Grand Ave.
Oakland, CA 94612
(510) 268-0572

Orange County Chapter
17500 Redhill Ave., Suite 240
Irvine, CA 92614
(949) 752-1680

*Southern California Chapter
2440 S. Sepulveda Blvd., Suite 115
Los Angeles, CA 90064
(310) 479-4456

San Diego Area Chapter
8840 Complex Dr., Suite 130
San Diego, CA 92123
(858) 974-8640

Silicon Valley Chapter
2589 Scott Blvd.
Santa Clara, CA 95050
(408) 988-7557

Central California Branch
Mountain Valley Chapter
1900 N. Gateway Blvd., #120
Fresno, CA 93727
(559) 252-2890

East County Branch Office
San Diego Area Chapter
1100 N. Magnolia, #E
El Cajon, CA 92020-1953
(619) 593-7790

Imperial Valley Branch
San Diego Area Chapter
P.O. Box 179
El Centro, CA 92244-0179
(760) 353-5432

North County Branch
San Diego Area Chapter
701 Palomar Airport Rd., 3rd Floor
Carlsbad, CA 92009
(760) 931-4766

Antelope/Santa Clarita Valley
    Branch Office
Southern California Chapter
23300 Cinema Dr., #275
Valencia, CA 91355
(805) 284-1655

Coachella Valley Branch Office
Southern California Chapter
73710 Fred Waring Dr., #103
Palm Desert, CA 92260
(760) 776-5740

Inland Empire Branch Office
Southern California Chapter
5 E. Citrus, Suite 107
Redlands, CA 92373
(909) 307-3388

Colorado
*Colorado Chapter
700 Broadway, Suite 808
Denver, CO 80203
(303) 831-0700
[Ms. Beverly Noyes, Ph.D., C.R.C.
    in Suite 810, National Director
    for Employment and Client
    Services (303) 813-6608]

Fort Collins Branch, Colorado
    Chapter
424 Pine, #104
Fort Collins, CO 80524
(970) 482-4807

Pueblo Branch
Colorado Chapter
803 W. 4th St., Suite E
Pueblo, CO 81003
(719) 545-8663

Western Slope Branch
Colorado Chapter
743 Horizon Court, #210
Grand Junction, CO 81506
(970) 241-9329

Connecticut
Greater Connecticut Chapter
705 N Mountain Rd., Suite G102
Newington, CT 06111
(860) 953-0601

Western Connecticut Chapter
One Selleck St., Suite 500
Norwalk, CT 06855
(203) 838-1033

Delaware
Delaware Chapter
Two Mill Rd., Suite 106
Wilmington, DE 19806
(302) 655-5610

Kent County Office, Delaware
    Chapter
606 Walker Rd.
Dover, DE 19901
(302) 734-8749

Southern Delaware Office
Delaware Chapter
Beebe Medical Ctr., c/o NMSS
424 Savannah Rd
Lewes, DE 19958-1462
(302) 645-1844

*District of Columbia
National Capital Chapter
2021 K St. NW, Suite 715
Washington, DC 20006
(202) 296-5363
[Project With Industry: Operation
    Job Match]

Florida
Mid-Florida Chapter
3659 Maguire Blvd., Suite 110
Orlando, FL 32803
(407) 896-3873

North Florida Chapter
9550 Regency Square Blvd., Suite 104
Jacksonville, FL 32225
(904) 725-6800

South Florida Chapter
5450 N.W. 33rd Ave., Suite 110
Fort Lauderdale, FL 33309
(954) 731-4224

Tampa Area Office, Mid-Florida
    Chapter
200 S. Hoover Blvd., Bldg 215,
    Suite 120
Tampa, FL 33609
(813) 287-2939

Georgia
Georgia Chapter
12 Perimeter Center E., Suite 1200
Atlanta, GA 30346
(770) 393-8833

Hawaii
Hawaii Division
418 Kuwili St., #105
Honolulu, HI 96817
(808) 532-0811

Idaho
Idaho Division
1674 Hill Rd., Suite 18
Boise, ID 83702
(208) 388-1998

Illinois
Greater Illinois Chapter
910 W. Van Buren St., 4th Floor
Chicago, IL 60607
(312) 421-4500

Greater Illinois Branch
Greater Illinois Chapter
206 N.E. Madison
Peoria, IL 61602
(309) 673-4448

Indiana
Indiana State Chapter
7301 Georgetown Rd., Suite112
Indianapolis, IN 46268
(317) 870-2500

Iowa
Iowa Chapter
2400 86th St., Suite 29
Urbandale, IA 50322
(515) 270-6337

Kansas
Mid-America Chapter
5442 Martway
Shawnee Mission, KS 66205
(913) 432-3926

South Central & Western Kansas
   Division
250 S. Laura
Wichita, KS 67211
(316) 264-1333

Eastern Kansas Branch
Mid-America Chapter
5350 SW 17th St.
Topeka, KS 66604
(913) 272-5292

Kentucky
Kentucky/Southeast Indiana Chapter
1169 Eastern Parkway, Suite 2266
Louisville, KY 40217

Louisiana
Louisiana Chapter
3616 S. I-10 Service Rd., Suite 101
Metairie, LA 70001
(504) 832-4013

Baton Rouge Unit, Louisiana
   Chapter
5319 Didesse Dr., Suite C
Baton Rouge, LA 70808
(225) 766-4348

Maine
Maine Chapter
P.O. Box 8730
Portland, ME 04104
(207) 761-5815

Maryland
Maryland Chapter
Hunt Valley Business Center
10946 Beaver Dam Rd, Suite E
Cockeysville, MD 21030
(410) 527-1770

Eastern Shore Area Branch
Maryland Chapter
207 Maryland Ave., Suite 4
Salisbury, MD 21801
(410) 543-0007

Southern Maryland Area Branch
Maryland Chapter
8338 Veterans Hghwy, #103-A
Millersville, MD 21108
(410) 987-3902

Tri County Branch
Maryland Chapter
15 E. Main St.
Westminster, MD 21157
(410) 840-9203

Western Maryland Area Branch
Maryland Chapter
119 E. Baltimore St., #A
Hagerstown, MD 21740
(301) 791-5754

Massachusetts

Central New England Chapter
101A First Ave., Suite 6
Waltham, MA 02451
(781) 890-4990

Southeastern Regional Office
Central New England Chapter
P.O. Box 329
Wareham, MA 02571-0329
(508) 291-2169

Western Region—Development
    Office
Central New England Chapter
P.O. Box 1463
Greenfield, MA 01302
(413) 659-0036

Western Region—Programs Office
Central New England Chapter
425 Union St.
West Springfield, MA 01089-4115
(413) 731-5362

Michigan

Michigan Chapter
26111 Evergreen, Suite 100
Southfield, MI 48076
(248) 350-0020

Eastern Region, Michigan Chapter
1312 Sugar Bush Ct.
Burton, MI 48509
(810) 742-5315

Western Michigan Region
Michigan Chapter
2020 Raybrook SE, Suite 204
Grand Rapid, MI 49546-7717
(616) 942-5505

Minnesota

Minnesota Chapter
200 12th Ave. S.
Minneapolis, MN 55415
(612) 335-7900

Northern Branch, Minnesota
    Chapter
707 Highway 33 S., Pinetree Plaza,
    #6
Cloquet, MN 55720
(218) 879-4540

Mississippi

Mississippi Division
145 Executive Dr., Suite 1
Madison, MS 39110
(601) 856-7575

Missouri

Gateway Area Chapter
1867 Lackland Hill Pkwy
Saint Louis, MO 63146
(314) 781-9020

Ozark Branch, Mid America
    Chapter
1675-1 E. Seminole
Springfield, MO 65804
(417) 882-8128

St. Joseph Branch
Mid-America Chapter
801 Faraon, Rm 238
St. Joseph, MO 64501
(816) 271-7560

Montana
Montana Division
1242 N 28th St., Suite 1003
Billings, MT 59101
(406) 252-9500

Nebraska
Nebraska Chapter
Community Health Plaza
7101 Newport Ave., Suite 203
Omaha, NE 68152
(402) 572-3190

Nevada
Great Basin Sierra Chapter
1201 Terminal Way, Suite 215
Reno, NV 89502
(775) 329-7180

Las Vegas Branch Office
Desert Southwest Chapter
6000 S. Eastern Ave., #5C
Las Vegas, NV 89119-5151
(702) 736-7272

New Hampshire
Northern Regional Office
Central New England Chapter
20 Commerce Park N, Suite 108
Bedford, NH 03110
(781) 890-4990

New Jersey
Greater North Jersey Chapter
1 Kalisa Way, Suite 205
Paramus, NJ 07652
(201) 967-5599

Mid-Jersey Chapter
1500 Lawrence Ave., 1st Floor
Asbury Park, NJ 07712
(732) 643-0010

New Mexico
Rio Grande Division
2021 Girard SE, #201
Albuquerque, NM 87106
(505) 244-0625

New York
Long Island Chapter
200 Parkway Dr. S., #101
Hauppauge, NY 11788
(516) 864-8337

Northeastern New York Chapter
9 Columbia Circle
Albany, NY 12203
(518) 464-0630

New York City Chapter
30 W 26th St., 9th Floor
New York, NY 10010
(212) 463-7787

Southern New York Chapter
11 Skyline Dr.
Hawthorne, NY 10532
(914) 345-3500

West New York/Northwest
   Pennsylvania Chapter
4245 Union Rd., Suite 108
Buffalo, NY 14225
(716) 634-2261

Upstate New York Chapter
1650 South Ave., Suite 100
Rochester, NY 14620
(716) 271-0801

Binghamton Branch Office
Upstate New York Chapter
457 State St.
Binghamton, NY 13901
(607) 724-5464

Syracuse Branch Office
Upstate New York Chapter
3532 James St., #104
Syracuse, NY 13206
(315) 431-9993

North Carolina
Central North Carolina Chapter
2211 W Meadowview Rd., Suite 30
Greensboro, NC 27407
(336) 299-4136

Eastern North Carolina Chapter
3101 Industrial Dr., Suite 210
Raleigh, NC 27609
(919) 834-0678

Mid Atlantic Chapter
9844 C Southern Pines Blvd.
Charlotte, NC 28273
(704) 525-2955

Central North Carolina Satellite
    Office
4265 Brownsboro Rd., Suite 150
Winston Salem, NC 27106-3425
(336) 759-2105

North Dakota
North Dakota Branch Office
Dakota Chapter
2801 Main Ave.
Fargo, ND 58103
(701) 235-2678

Ohio
Northeast Ohio Chapter/Greater
    Cleveland Branch
The Hanna Building
1422 Euclid Ave., Suite 333
Cleveland, OH 44115
    (614) 459-2220

Mid-Ohio Chapter
1550 Old Henderson Rd, W-101
Columbus, OH 43220
(216) 696-8220

Northwest Ohio Chapter
415 Tomahawk Dr.
Maumee, OH 43537
(419) 897-9533

Southwest Ohio/North Kentucky
    Chapter
4460 Lake Forest Dr., Suite 236
Cincinnati, OH 45242
(513) 769-4400

Western Ohio Chapter
The Woolpert Building
409 E. Monument, Suite 101
Dayton, OH 45402
(937) 461-5232

*Greater Akron/Canton Branch
Northeast Ohio Chapter
520 S. Main St., Suite 2501
Akron, OH 44311
(330) 434-3411

Oklahoma
Oklahoma Chapter
4606 E. 67th St., Suite 103
Tulsa, OK 74136
(918) 488-0882

Oregon
Oregon Chapter
1650 NW Front Ave., Suite 190
Portland, OR 97209
(503) 223-9511

Pennsylvania
Allegheny District Chapter
1040 Fifth Ave., 2nd Floor
Pittsburgh, PA 15219
(412) 261-6347

Central Pennsylvania Chapter
2209 Forest Hills Dr., #18
Harrisburg, PA 17112
(717) 652-2108

Greater Delaware Valley Chapter
1 Reed St.
Philadelphia, PA 19147
(215) 271-2400

Keystone Branch
Allegheny District Chapter
506 3rd Ave.
Duncansville, PA 16635
(814) 696-1017

North Central Pennsylvania Branch
Central Pennsylvania Chapter
175 Pine St.
Williamsport, PA 17701
(717) 326-3751

Northeastern Branch
Central Pennsylvania Chapter
P.O. Box 86
West Pittson, PA 18643
(717) 654-0838

Southeastern Branch
Central Pennsylvania Chapter
117 D South West End Ave.
Lancaster, PA 17603
(717) 397-1481

Lehigh Valley Branch
Greater Delaware Valley Chapter
1259 S. Cedar Crest Blvd., #313
Allentown, PA 18103
(610) 78-9450

Reading Area Branch Office
Greater Delaware Valley Chapter
509A Madison Ave.
Reading, PA 19605
(610) 939-9088

Rhode Island
Rhode Island Chapter
205 Hallene Rd., Suite 209
Warwick, RI 02886
(401) 738-8383

South Carolina
South Carolina Regional Office
Mid-Atlantic Chapter
2711 Middleburg Dr., #105
Columbia, SC 29204
(803) 799-7848

South Dakota
Dakota Chapter
1000 E. 41st St.
Sioux Falls, SD 57105
(605) 336-7017

Tennessee

Mid-South Chapter
6685 Quince Rd., Suite 124
Memphis, TN 38119
(901) 755-4900

Middle Tennessee Chapter
4219 Hillsboro Rd., Suite 306
Nashville, TN 37215
(615) 269-9055

Southeast Tennessee/North Georgia
   Chapter
5720 Uptain Rd., Suite 4800
Chattanooga, TN 37411
(423) 954-9700

East Tennessee Regional Office
Mid-Atlantic Chapter
P.O. Box 52068
Knoxville, TN 37950-2068
(423) 558-8686

Texas

Lone Star Chapter
2211 Norfolk, Suite 825
Houston, TX 77098
(713) 526-8967

North Texas Chapter
8750 N Central Expressway,
   Suite 1030
Dallas, TX 75231
(214) 373-1400

North Central Texas Chapter
2501 Parkview Dr., Suite 550
Fort Worth, TX 76102
(817) 877-1222

Panhandle Chapter
6222 Canyon Dr.
Amarillo, TX 79109
(806) 468-7500

West Texas Division Chapter
1031 Andrews Hwy, Suite 201
Midland, TX 79701
(915) 522-2077

Central Texas Branch, Lone Star
1601 Rio Grande, #445
Austin, TX 78701
(512) 495-9901

San Antonio Branch
Lone Star Chapter
140 Heimer, #195
San Antonio, TX 78232
(210) 494-5531

Utah

Utah State Chapter
2995 SW Temple, Suite C
Salt Lake City, UT 84115
(801) 493-0113

Vermont

Vermont Division
100 Dorset St., Suite 12
South Burlington, VT 05403

Virginia

Blue Ridge Chapter
1 Morton Dr., Suite 106
Charlottesville, VA 22903
(804) 971-8010

Central Virginia Chapter
1301 N Hamilton St., Suite 108
Richmond, VA 23230
(804) 353-5008

Hampton Roads Chapter
405 S. Parliament Dr., Suite 105
Virginia Beach, VA 23462
(757) 490-9627

Roanoke Branch, Blue Ridge
    Chapter
3959 Electric Rd. SW, #310
Roanoke, VA 24018
(540) 776-0985

Washington

Greater Washington Chapter
192 Nickerson St., Suite 100
Seattle, WA 98109
(206) 284-4236

Inland Northwest Chapter
818 E. Sharp
Spokane, WA 99202
(509) 482-2022

Central Washington Branch Office
Greater Washington Chapter
P.O. Box 1093
Yakima, WA 98907
(509) 248-2350

West Virginia

West Virginia Chapter
111 Hale St.
Charleston, WV 25301
(304) 343-5152

Wisconsin

Wisconsin Chapter
W223 N608 Saratoga Dr., Suite 110
Waukesha, WI 53186
(262) 547-8999

Wyoming

341 East E., Suite 100
Casper, WY 82602
(307) 234-2340

About the Paralyzed Veterans of America (PVA)

Organized following World War II, PVA is a nonprofit organization dedicated to serving the needs of its members—all of whom have catastrophic paralysis caused by spinal cord injury or disease including multiple sclerosis. Since its inception, PVA has been in the forefront of improving health care, rehabilitation, and access to society for paralyzed veterans. PVA also supports initiatives designed to help all veterans and all Americans with disabilities. Today, PVA is a dynamic, broad-based organization with more than 40 chapters and subchapters and 58 national service offices nationwide. Since its founding, PVA activities and programs have expanded dramatically in size and scope, from veterans benefits to rehabilitation engineering, from medical research to legislative action, from public education to wheelchair sports. PVA's key objective is to take those actions that will help veterans with spinal cord dysfunction restore their physical capabilities and quality of life as closely as possible to those of the nondisabled population. PVA's national office may be reached at 1-800-424-8200 or by visiting www.pva.org. The major chapters are listed below while information regarding the subchapters may be found by calling or visiting the PVA website.

Harlon Cauthron
President
Arizona PVA
1016 N. 32nd Street, #4
Phoenix, AZ 85008
(602) 244-9168

Bruce Kent
President
Bayou Gulf States PVA
1808 19th Street
Gulfport, MS 39501
(228) 868-6976

Don Hyslop
President
Cal-Diego PVA
3350 LaJolla Village Drive,
    Suite 1A-118
San Diego, CA 92161
(858) 450-1443

Gary Rudolph
President
Central Florida PVA
2711 South Design Court
Sanford, FL 32773
(407) 328-7041

Angelo Bianco
President
Eastern PVA
75-20 Astoria Boulevard
Jackson Heights, NY 11370-1177
(718) 803-3782

James Griffith
President
Bay Area & Western PVA
3801 Miranda Ave., Rm A1-219
Mailing Code 816
Palo Alto, CA 94304
(650) 855-9030

Walter Ward
President
Buckeye PVA
10545 Wyndtree Drive
Concord, OH 44077
(216) 731-1017

Ronald Amador
President
California PVA
5901 E. Seventh Street,
    Bldg 122 F-130
Long Beach, CA 90822
(562) 494-5713

Ronald Hoskins, Sr.
President
Delaware-Maryland PVA
1658 Bondsville Road
Dowington, PA 19335
(302) 368-4898

Angus Farnum
President
Florida Gulf Coast PVA
121 West 122nd Avenue
Tampa, FL 33612
(813) 935-6540

David Monson
President
Florida PVA
6200 N. Andrews Avenue
Ft. Lauderdale, FL 33309
(954) 771-7822

William Blow
President
Great Plains PVA
7612 Maple Street
Omaha, NE 68134-6502
(402) 398-1422

James Elliott
President
Kentucky-Indiana PVA
1030 Goss Avenue
Louisville, KY 40217-1236
(502) 635-6539

Jack Hasenyager
President
Lone Star PVA
3925 Forest Lane
Garland, TX 75042
(972) 276-5252

Robert Cornsilk
President
Mid-America PVA
Route 4, Box 1280
Stilwell, OK 74060
(405) 721-7168
(901) 527-3018

Gene Crayton
President
Gateway PVA
9535 Lackland Road
St. Louis, MO 63114
(314) 427-0393

Jon Schneider
President
Iowa PVA
3703 1/2 Douglas Avenue
Des Moines, IA 50310
(515) 277-4782

Thomas Matthews, Jr.
President
Keystone PVA
203 Butler Street
Pittsburgh, PA 15223-2006
(412) 784-9320

James Jachim
President
Michigan PVA
40550 Grand River Avenue
Novi, MI 48375
(248) 476-9000

Aubrey Crockett
President
Mid-South PVA
Memphis VAMC (817)
1030 Jefferson Avenue, Room 2D100
Memphis, TN 38104

Oliver Skov
President
Minnesota PVA
1 Veteran Drive, 4J-117
Minneapolis, MN 55417
(612) 725-2263

Larry Callaghan
President
New England PVA
3 Highland Lake Drive
Norfolk, MA 02056
(508) 660-1181

Gary Pearson
President
Northwest PVA
616 SW 152nd, Suite B
Burien, WA 98166
(206) 241-1843

James Torres
President
Puerto Rico PVA
63 Calle Rey Melchor Street
Bonneville Valley Townhouse
Caguas, PR 00725
(787) 757-6465

Frank Homesley
President
Texas PVA
Route 1, Box 117
Georgetown, TX 78626
(713) 520-8782

James Sack
President
Mountain States PVA
1734 Dahlia Street
Denver, CO 80220
(603) 322-4402

Michael Olson
President
North Central PVA
209 North Garfield
Sioux Falls, SD 57104-5601
(605) 336-0494

Roger Robinson
President
Oregon PVA
13863 Doerfler Road
Silverton, OR 97381
(503) 362-7998

Charles Littleton
President
Southeastern PVA
4010 Deans Bridge Road
Hephzibah, GA 30815
(706) 796-6301

James Derrico
President
Vaughan PVA
2153 Hidden Valley Drive
Naperville, IL 60563
(630) 579-0775

John Jackson
President
Virginia - Mid-Atlantic PVA
11620 Busy Street
Richmond, VA 23236
(804) 378-0017

Phillip Rosenberg
President
Wisconsin PVA
6069 N. Jean Nicholet
Glendale, WI 53217
(414) 475-7792

Randy Pleva
President
West Virginia PVA
336 Campbells Creek Drive
Charleston, WV 25306
(304) 925-9352

Ron Gattas
President
Zia PVA
912 Chama NE
Albuquerque, NM 87110
(505) 247-4381

Index

Note: Boldface numbers indicate illustrations.